FIGHTING BACK:

HOW TO PROTECT YOURSELF

AGAINST THE "FOOD BUG"

AND REPORT

FOOD POISONING HAZARDS

Michael H. Doom R.E.H.S.
Registered Environmental Health Specialist

Illustrations and Cover by Charles J. Moore

First Edition - 1992

Published By
M&C Publishing
8121 Manchester Blvd., #594A
Los Angeles, CA 90293

Printed in the United States

First Edition 1992

Library of Congress Catalog Number: 91-90127

ISBN 0-9628988-5-6

Introduction

Chances are that at least once in your life you have been food poisoned and knew it, but there have probably been plenty of times which you either can't recall or you passed it off as "the flu". Food poisoning or food-borne illness is much more common and serious than the general population realizes. In fact, becoming ill or dying from eating food contaminated with microorganisms or germs is the greatest food safety risk. It's higher than pesticide risks, environmental contaminants, nutritional imbalances, food additives and natural toxicants. 90% of the diseases or illnesses associated with food are caused by microorganism contamination. Microorganisms are everywhere. Even the cleanest employee, freshest food or the most immaculate kitchen has some microorganisms.

The United States Department of Agriculture estimates that roughly 7 million cases of food poisoning occur each year in the U.S. The actual number of food-borne illness cases is most likely much higher since approximately only 1-5% of food poisonings are reported. Some estimates approximate the total number of food poisoning episodes or cases which occur, each year in the U.S., as high as 81 million.

A sadder statistic is the approximately 9,000 deaths resulting from food poisoning in the U.S. each year. The highest incidence of death due to food poisoning occurs in children, elderly and people who are chronically ill or with weakened immune systems, such as Aids, cancer and kidney disease patients. Just because you're healthy doesn't mean you can't die from food poisoning. There have been many reported cases of young healthy people not surviving a food poisoning illness. Genetic differences make some persons more susceptible than others. Chronic antibiotic use or pregnancy may also be a risk factor. Infants have incompletely developed immune systems.

Surprisingly, most food-borne illnesses are caused by improper food handling in the home. The misconception that food poisoning is more likely to occur at commercial establishments is due to the fact that the only time most people hear about food

1

poisonings is when a large number of people have become ill or have died from eating the same food at some large gathering or a restaurant. The only other way food poisoning gets in the news is through a much-publicized government recall of a commercial product.

Thanks to strict standards and government inspections within the food industry, Americans generally enjoy the safest, most nutritious food, and most abundant food supply in the world. There are many theories to explain why food-borne illness still occurs and has been on the rise for the past 15 years.

One reason is a general lack of knowledge (which this author hopes to remedy), among recent newcomers to America, of basic food sanitation practices. Other cultures have different sanitation practices and in many cases these are more hazardous to ones health than those normally practiced in the United States.

Another reason for the occurrence and increase in food-borne illness might have to do with mass production or changes in production in the food processing and production industries, which allows for greater spread of contamination. Still other reasons might be the decrease in frequency, quality or overall lack of inspections in certain areas and in certain industries. I'm sure there are other theories or reasons and the cause of the increase is probably a combination of all of them.

These statistics and theories are not meant to instill fear or paranoia in anyone. My main purpose in writing this book is to educate people about a subject which I believe is not very well understood or recognized. This book explains general practices and guidelines to help you avoid food-borne illness and to recognize common Health and Safety Code violations.

I have worked for more than four years as a Environmental Health Specialist for the County of Los Angeles, and during those years I have seen how much harm a little ignorance on this subject can do.

By learning this information and putting it into practice, I believe you can greatly reduce the risk of food-borne illness for you, your family and your friends.

I have divided this book into sections according to different situations you will probably come across every week, if not every day. The first section concerns dining out, including all types of restaurants, delicatessens, bakeries, ice cream parlors, street vendors, and catering trucks. The second section concerns food markets and what you should be looking out for while shopping at the grocery store. The third section concerns outdoor and indoor picnics, carnivals, fairs, and barbecues. The fourth section deals with home food preparation safety. In the last section I explain how to report food-borne illness and any violations you've observed to your local Health Department.

All references to laws in this book come directly from the California State Health and Safety Code which is enforced throughout the State of California. All states, most counties and some cities have their own set or version of Health and Safety Codes which are fairly similar throughout the United States. As a violation of the law food poisoning can be, and in most cases should be, reported to your local Health Department to protect others from harm in the future.

FOOD POISONING HAZARDS

The information in this book reflects California Health and Safety Law and recommendations from different sources, including but not limited to the U.S. Department of Agriculture, and draws upon as well the author's own knowledge and experience. This book is not intended as a substitute for medical advice of physicians. The reader should regularly consult with a physician in matters relating to his or her health and particularly in respect to any symptoms which might require diagnosis or medical attention. Every reader must consult with his or her physician before starting or stopping any medication and before implementing any other form of therapy or recommendation in this book. More importantly, any side effects should be immediately reported to a trained physician.

TABLE OF CONTENTS

What you, the consumer, should be on the lookout for whenever you eat out. Find out what clues health inspectors look for. Even the nicest establishment can pose a threat to your health!

A complete explanation of what standards apply to various types of food markets and how they protect your health.

Chapter 1
The Dining Out Experience

What should you, as a consumer, look out for that could possibly warn yourself that you or others could get sick, or just plain disgusted, by eating at an establishment? Since there are a few different types of dining-out businesses, I have divided this section into three basic categories: Restaurants; Catering Trucks; and Sidewalk or Street Vendors. I'll start first with the most common dining experience for many people - the Restaurant.

RESTAURANTS

For the purpose of this text I am including any permanently located business where food is being stored and prepared on the premises, and served, retail to customers as a restaurant.

This definition should include all sit down, or drive through restaurants, delicatessens, bakeries, ice cream parlors, cafeterias, or any other commercial or institutional kitchen. Many food markets also have delis, bakeries, and/or meat markets, all of which do some food preparation and therefore fall under the same guidelines as a restaurant in the Health and Safety Code.

The Health and Safety Code defines food preparation as "packaging processing, assembling, portioning, or any operation which changes the form, flavor, or consistency of food, but does not include trimming of produce."

What specifically should you be aware of when judging a restaurant? Divide the average restaurant into five areas and analyze each of them, starting with (a) the outside surrounding grounds, then (b) the kitchen and food preparation areas, followed by (c) the dining areas, (d) the food itself, and, finally, (e) the restrooms. You need to use all your senses, especially sight, smell, and taste.

(a) EXTERIOR

When you first drive or walk up to a restaurant you should take note of the trash area and surrounding grounds because this can be a pretty good indication of the condition of the kitchen just inside. Is there an unpleasant odor? Are the trash containers open with flies flying in and out? Is the trash being stored in tied, sealed plastic bags? Is the trash overflowing from the containers or deposited on the ground? Is there an accumulation of other rubbish, such as old equipment, mattresses or other cluttered junk, on the outside premises, which might allow rat or mouse refuge? These conditions might be considered minor since they are outside the restaurant, but this can be, from my experience as a health inspector, a good indication of the sanitation practices and general upkeep of the restaurant kitchen.

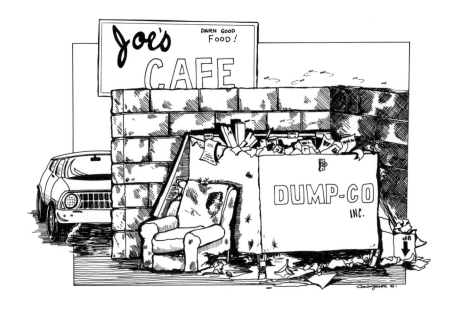

Unkept trash areas or outside grounds also may result in flies, rats, mice, and cockroaches - all of which are significant public health problems, and they can make their way inside the restaurant.

(b) *FOOD PREPARATION AREAS*

If you are standing in line and ordering from the counter, or are near doorways or windows which let you see into the kitchen area, there are a number of things you can look for. You can even ask to see the kitchen. The worst the manager can say is no, which just gives you another signal to be suspicious. If he says yes, then open your eyes and scrutinize. Go slow, look carefully and sniff the air and the food.

FOOD POISONING HAZARDS

FOOD HANDLERS

Look to see if the food handlers are wearing clean clothing, aprons, etc., and some kind of adequate hair restraint - either a hat or hair net - to hold all of their hair in place. Hair may contain germs that can cause illness if they get into your food, as I'll describe a little later. Food handlers should be wearing clean aprons and they should not wipe their hands on the aprons. Aprons must be changed whenever they become too soiled.

If the food handlers are wearing gloves take that as a good sign. Gloves are generally not required and most of the time you will not see cooks or kitchen staff with gloves on. This is unfortunate since a very large number of food-borne illnesses are spread by hand-to-food contact. Gloves are not a guarantee against food contamination. They can become contaminated and contaminate your food. Gloves are not a substitute for washing the hands. Fingernails of food handlers must be kept clean, cut short and well manicured. A utensil should be used as much as possible, such as in the making of salads and soups. Humans are the number one cause of food contamination and it comes from the hands.

Employees serving food should always be using tongs, forks or spoons, rather than their hands.

You should also know that it is not illegal for employees to handle food and money without washing their hands in between. All currency paper printed in the United States contains fungicidal agents which have germicidal characteristics, and retains their effectiveness throughout the life of the currency in circulation. The ink used on paper money also contains ingredients which inhibit the growth of bacteria. Surveys of both paper currency and metal coins, revealed low numbers of germs. All of this means that money is not any dirtier than the average handled utensil, and although employees who come in contact with food and food contact surfaces must wash their hands as often as necessary to keep them clean, it is not necessary that they wash their hands each time they handle money.

Makeup, perfume and jewelry can also contaminate your food and should be kept to a minimum on all food handlers.

Other bad habits to look for while checking out the food handlers (which includes servers, as well) are any use of tobacco, spitting, rubbing or picking the nose, ears, pimples or boils, licking their fingers, or eating while working or just eating or chewing gum in the kitchen area. All of these habits can potentially contaminate your food with hazardous germs. Hands can and do pick up bacteria - the most common food poisoning microorganism or germ. There is also the possibility of expectorating germs while eating food or chewing. The saliva, nasal discharges, ears and skin (especially infections) of all of us, contain large numbers of bacteria which are normally harmless until given the proper environment to reproduce to very large numbers. In large numbers they may become dangerous enough to cause illness or infection, to yourself or others. I will describe what the proper environment for food poisoning microorganisms is a little later in this chapter.

Smoking, or any form of tobacco use, by employees is definitely not allowed in any area where food is prepared, served, or stored, or utensils are cleaned or stored, for a number of important reasons: 1. A person smoking can easily pick up saliva on his or her hands by touching his mouth or touching the cigarette that just came from the mouth. This saliva is then passed on to your food as soon as this food handler touches it; 2. The ashes and cigarette butts left behind may be dropped or spilled and thereby mixed into your food.

One last thing to notice about the food handlers is their general health. Any food handlers, including servers, who appear ill should definitely not be anywhere near food preparation or storage areas. Take note of any general symptoms of a cold, or flu, such as coughing, sniffling, etc. These common illnesses are spread very easily, and food makes a very good vehicle. If you see an ill employee working around food, you should definitely think twice about eating at this establishment. In fact, you should contact your local Health Department right away about such a situation.

CLEANLINESS

Other things to look for if you have a view of the kitchen include the overall cleanliness. Does the floor, walls, ceiling, shelves, equipment, etc., have an accumulation of dust, dirt, grease, food particles, crumbs or trash? All surfaces in a kitchen and food storage area must be kept very clean. There should not be any over accumulations of trash or junk - including unused equipment, tools, etc. stored in these areas. Everything should be neat and well organized. Accumulations of dust, dirt, grease, food particles or trash or general uncleanliness attract and maintain vermin (mice, rats, cockroaches, flies and other insects and animals) and microorganisms.

All food establishments must be maintained and operated so as to prevent the entrance and harborage of vermin. The establishment should never have mice, rats, flies, cockroaches or other insects, spiders, etc. Vermin are strictly illegal in all areas of the establishment which includes the kitchen, food or equipment storage areas, restrooms, customer service and seating areas, and trash storage areas. They're illegal not just because they are unsightly and can get into your food, but mainly because they may carry numerous diseases and they may transmit those diseases onto us by coming in contact with our food or food contact surfaces, such as cutting boards, utensils, plates, glasses, etc.

All walls, ceilings, floors, shelves, and equipment must not only be kept clean but also smooth, easily cleanable and maintained in good repair. There should be no peeling of paint, plaster, rust accumulation, or any damaged equipment. Peeling paint, plaster or other materials are considered hazardous and can possibly make their way into your food. All equipment, such as stoves and refrigerators must be maintained in good working order so the equipment will be used and cleaned regularly.

Also look for possible contamination of food, food-contact surfaces, equipment, or utensils, by overhead leakage, poisonous chemical substance or even sewage from a backed up drain. Overhead leakage is any water, including rain water, or any substance leaking from equipment, pipes, ceiling, etc., which contacts and therefore contaminates, food, food-contact surfaces or utensils. Any water, other than the water coming from a faucet, is considered potentially hazardous and should not come in contact with food or food-contact surfaces.

Poisonous substances include insecticides, rodenticides, cleaning chemicals and so on. These chemical substances should never be stored in a manner that can potentially contaminate food. They should be stored in an enclosed cabinet, closet or room containing only chemical substances and no food products. They should never be stored on tables or shelves in the kitchen and must always be stored in labeled containers and maintained in an organized manner.

A stopped up sink, floor drain or toilet is not uncommon in a busy restaurant. Immediate efforts must be made by the restaurant employees or management to prevent any food contamination and to have the sink, or toilet, drain repaired at

15

once. The Health Department may order the establishment to close if the back up is not repaired immediately and all contaminated surfaces are not thoroughly cleaned and sanitized. The health inspector will make the judgement on whether or not to close the restaurant.

VERMIN

Vermin in a food establishment is a very serious problem and a public health danger, and should be immediately reported to your local Health Department. A heavy infestation of some vermin, such as cockroaches and rodents, will sometimes give the restaurant a recognizable musty odor. If you detect this odor, be wary about eating there and look for other clues. A restaurant should always smell clean and of fresh food. Anything else could mean something is wrong.

Many people, including the restaurant operators believe vermin are in every restaurant and food establishment, and are as much a part of the restaurant as the customers. These people believe that you can never completely get rid of vermin. Both of these statements are, of course, false. All types of restaurants, even the newest, nicest, most expensive, elegant restaurant can become infested with vermin. But, with good sanitation practices and thorough rodent and insect proofing, extermination and insecticide treatment, one can eliminate and prevent infestations. If a restaurant can not fully eliminate the vermin it is their own fault. The restaurant should be closed either voluntarily or by order of the Health Department.

Vermin infestations are fairly common in food establishments and when observed by an inspector orders are immediately written up to eliminate the infestation. Most restaurants will comply. Those that don't may have their health permit suspended or revoked and must therefore close, or they are taken to court for criminal prosecution, or both.

In many older buildings, vermin can be more difficult to eliminate. The reason for this is that there are many more hiding spaces for vermin in older buildings which are not easily accessible. There may also be other nonfood businesses adjacent to or in the same building, which are doing little or nothing to help eliminate the vermin. Insects, such as cockroaches, can find other things to eat when our food or garbage is not available. So what is the solution to these problems? Here's a few answers.

Newer buildings are designed and built to exclude and prevent vermin from settling in (vermin harborage) with fewer hiding spaces and easier access to all areas of the building. This is not to say that in older buildings one can never eliminate the vermin. The Health Inspector will work with the restaurant operator to upgrade the building and eliminate all those hiding places. Also, the inspector will show the operator how to improve general sanitation practices and help set up programs for overall food safety and sanitation. The inspector can also issue orders to any nonfood businesses to eliminate vermin infestations.

There is no excuse for a vermin infestation and the restaurant operator must eliminate the vermin to stay in business. The Health Inspector will close the restaurant and/or filing criminal charges if the operator fails to eliminate all vermin from his or her establishment. There is no middle ground when it comes to public health and safety, especially in a food establishment.

FOOD POISONING HAZARDS

ANIMALS

Live animals and birds are also not allowed in a restaurant. Dogs used by the blind, signal dogs and service dogs are exempt only for the customer service area. Aquariums and aviaries are also allowed if they are enclosed and do not create a public health problem. Animals may carry vermin and disease-causing organisms, as well as dirt and filth. You should, therefore, never see them in a food establishment, with the exception of those special cases just described. If animals are kept outside they must be kept a certain distance away from the building. This distance varies between different local Health Department Codes.

PICTORIAL PUZZLE #1

The kitchen pictured below gives you a chance to apply some of the information I have given you concerning health hazards. There are fourteen separate potential health hazards depicted here. Can you identify all of them? Look closely, jot down your list, and then check your answers against those provided at the back of this book on page 123. And, yes, I've seen all of these violations in restaurants I've inspected, sometimes all at once!

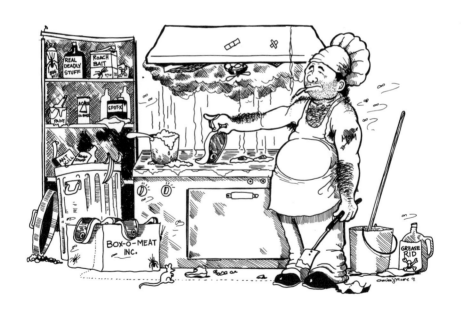

(c) *DINING AREAS*

If you do not have a view of the kitchen area there are other clues to look for, which could indicate that this is an unhealthful place to eat.

While waiting for your waiter or waitress to take your order or deliver your food there are a few things you should take note of. Check over your silverware, glasses, cups, dishes and even your table, to be sure that they are clean and in good condition. They should not be rusting, dirty, chipped or cracked. The chipped glass or plate can not only injure you but also consider this: Where did the chipped piece end up? Hopefully not in the food you're about to eat. Also, chipped or cracked dishes and glassware are difficult to clean.

Remember, you should not see vermin anywhere in a restaurant, including the customer seating and service areas. There is the possibility of finding a dead insect. This doesn't mean the restaurant presently has a problem with vermin, except, possibly, if it's in your food. They could have had a problem in the past and have exterminated and already eliminated the problem. Ask your server or the manager if they have a vermin problem and what they're doing or have done to eliminate it. Whatever the case, if you still feel safe eating at this establishment tell the server to remove the insect and have the surface cleaned right away.

Your waiter or waitress, just as the employees in the kitchen area, must be wearing clean outer garments, have some type of adequate hair restraint and not appear to be ill. Also, your server's finger nails should be trimmed short and clean.

The customer seating and service areas always look neater and cleaner than the kitchen and back storage areas. You, have to look for little subtle clues, such as dirt or dust on the fans or window sills. All hard to reach places in a restaurant should be kept clean.

(d) *FOOD*

The examination of your food, once you've received it, is very important in avoiding food poisoning. The consumption of food and drink is, of course, the final route a food-borne illness follows. I'm going to describe for you some basic tips to remember prior to and during consumption of your food.

FOOD TEMPERATURE

I'll start first with food temperatures. A basic rule of thumb to always remember for proper, safe temperature of your food is that if it is supposed to be hot or cold, it had better be hot or cold and not somewhere in between. This may sound pretty simple but it is also very important.

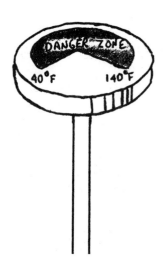

For meals which are supposed to be served hot, the simple test is that the food should not only feel very hot to the touch, but it should be steaming as well. This rule goes for both food that is on display, such as at a buffet-type setting, and when a server brings the food to you. Hot foods must be maintained at 140°F, though 165°F or even higher is a little safer. It's a good idea to familiarize your senses with this temperature by testing yourself at home, using a probe-type thermometer to measure the temperature of some food, and then remember how hot it feels to the touch when you feel or bite into it. You can buy a probe thermometer at any kitchen supply store or maybe your local grocery or hardware store.

For cold foods, it might be a little harder to sense that the food is at or below the maximum legal refrigeration temperature of 45°F, (40°F or below is safer). Again, you should familiarize yourself with this temperature at home. If the food is supposed to be cold it should not feel like room temperature or warmer and you should definitely feel some sensation of coldness when you touch or bite into it. Since there aren't many foods served at room temperature, and supposed to be at that temperature, I believe this is a good rule to practice.

Maintaining proper food temperatures is extremely important. Maintaining potentially hazardous foods at properly hot (165°F and above) or cold (40-45°F or below) temperatures is essential in avoiding the most common food poisonings. This temperature range, between 45° and 140°F, is called the food temperature danger zone, and the main objective in a good food establishment is to maintain food outside this range and when passing through this range, as in heating or cooling, food must pass through as quickly as possible.

Many, if not most, food poisoning investigations, performed after a food poisoning complaint, conclude that there was some violation in temperature control of the food. In fact, a 1982 annual summary survey, by the Centers for Disease Control, showed that improper holding temperature was by far the most common factor contributing to bacteria food-borne disease outbreaks. In the survey, contributing factors for each outbreak were broken down as follows:

Contributing factor:	Proportion of total outbreaks:
1. Improper holding temperature	67.37 %
2. Inadequate cooking	31.50 %
3. Poor personal hygiene	23.16 %
4. Contaminated equipment	13.68 %
5. Food from unsafe sources	10.53 %
Other	11.58 %

FOOD POISONING HAZARDS

(It should be noted that there were more than one contributing factor in some outbreaks, so the total of all the percentages is more than 100%.)

POTENTIALLY HAZARDOUS & PERISHABLE FOODS

Some background information on potentially hazardous and perishable foods is in order to give you some insight into what common types of foods can cause illness, and under what conditions.

All potentially hazardous foods are perishable, but not all perishable foods are potentially hazardous. Does that sound confusing? Perishable food, depending on how much time elapses - weeks, months, years - can pretty much include all food. Potentially hazardous foods not only spoil much faster than other perishable foods, but they can support microorganisms which can very readily cause illness.

Potentially hazardous food, as defined in the California Health and Safety Code, is "food capable of supporting rapid and progressive growth of microorganisms that may cause food infections or food intoxications." Food intoxication is caused by microorganisms which, under the right conditions, produce a toxin, or poisonous substance, capable of causing illness or death. Food infection results when the food contains enough microorganisms which, after being ingested, produce toxins or toxic effects that cause illness or death.

Potentially hazardous foods are really just foods which can readily cause illness if handled or stored improperly. There are a number of ways to handle or store food improperly. Improper temperature is one of the most important ones and the easiest one to check on if you aren't able to check the others.

SAFER FOODS

Not all foods are potentially hazardous, and in fact, probably the majority of food we buy in the market would not be considered potentially hazardous in the state in which they're bought and sold. Those foods which are not considered potentially hazardous fall into one or more of three conditions which generally inhibit or slow microorganism growth.

HIGH ACIDITY

Foods which are more on the acidic side (a pH of 4.6 or lower) are not considered potentially hazardous and include such foods as some types of pickles, certain processed meats, salad dressings, mayonnaise and many sauces. Most of these foods have either vinegar, lemon juice, acetic acid or other acidic substance in the ingredients which you can read on the label. Many of these products should be maintained refrigerated, even though they're not potentially hazardous, in order to maintain consistency and freshness. The label should tell you if this is the case.

LOW WATER CONTENT

A second condition is the amount of water in the food. Foods which have a free water content of 85% or lower are not considered potentially hazardous. This includes most dry foods, such as cereals, nuts, uncooked rice, most bakery products, sugar, flour, honey, dried meats, jams and jellies, dried fruit, chocolate, other candies, etc., which do not contain enough water to support rapid microorganism growth. Heavy salting of foods, such as fish and meats, also lowers the free water content in the food, thereby inhibiting or slowing microorganism growth.

Raw fruits, rice, pastas, and vegetables are generally safe at room temperature until the are processed or cooked. Once they are cut up, cooked or processed, they become exposed to possible contamination. Since many fruits and vegetables are not protected by one of the "safe" conditions we are considering, they can then become potentially hazardous.

Desserts and bakery products may be potentially hazardous, depending on their ingredients. Desserts containing dairy products and/or eggs which are creamy or moist and not on the acidic side must be refrigerated. Many bakery products contain egg- or milk-based fillings and must also be refrigerated.

Most breads, cookies, donuts, certain cakes and the like, do not contain enough water to support rapid microorganism growth and do not have to be refrigerated. However, they are perishable, since they will spoil after a week or more of storage.

PROPER CONTAINMENT

The third condition is proper containment of foods. Potentially hazardous foods do not include food products in hermetically sealed containers processed to prevent spoilage. This includes most commercially canned and bottled foods as well as other packages which, when sealed airtight, can be maintained at room temperature because of special packaging processes. When opened, though, most probably should be refrigerated or heated soon to prevent microorganism growth. The container label will say most of the time if it should be kept refrigerated.

POTENTIALLY HAZARDOUS FOODS

Now that I've described what's generally not considered potentially hazardous, let me give you a general idea of what is considered potentially hazardous:

MEAT, FISH AND POULTRY

All types of meats, fish and sea foods and land animal products, including beef, pork, chicken, duck, turkey and wild game are considered potentially hazardous unless they are processed in such a manner as to fall into one of those three "safe" conditions just described.

Fish, and all other animal sea food products, such as shellfish, squid, octopus and other mollusks, in their raw or partially cooked state, which is not too uncommon in many restaurants are just as dangerous as poultry and other meats. It is a widely accepted fact that there is a much greater chance of becoming ill or dying from eating raw or partially cooked seafood, meats and other potentially hazardous foods, than if you eat them thoroughly cooked. The simple reason behind this fact is that thorough cooking kills most common food poisoning microorganisms and parasites.

Seafood has become much more of a concern the last few years because of the increasing popularity of eating it in the raw state. Raw seafood is more of concern because of the increased chance of it being contaminated. The increase is theorized to be due, at least in part, to an increase in pollution in the waters in which they may have been taken from. *Hepatitis* and *salmonellosis* are two more common illnesses associated with eating raw seafood and, since the organisms which cause these illness are fairly common in sewage-polluted waters, it is one strong possibility. There is, of course, also the chance of becoming contaminated somewhere along the handling and processing chain, which can be quite long for fish and seafood products. My advice then is to always be sure your seafood (just as your poultry or beef) is thoroughly cooked. Also, whenever possible, find out if the restaurant has a policy of obtaining its seafood only from approved, reputable sources.

Unfortunately, thorough cooking doesn't <u>always</u> protect you from tainted seafood. Scombroid or histamine poisoning is caused by fish such as tuna or mackerel that has not been properly refrigerated before being cooked. A sharp, peppery or metallic taste should be a warning of this danger. Since the illness is caused by the toxins produced by the microorganisms and not the organisms themselves, no amount of cooking will destroy the poison. The only way to protect yourself from this type of food poisoning is to throw out the tainted fish.

Poultry - chicken, duck, turkey - has also become more of a concern over the past few years because of its potential for causing food-borne illness, and also its large increase in popularity. Many restaurants serve only, or mainly, chicken dishes, and it seems just about every restaurant has at least one chicken dish on the menu. So why does poultry have a high potential for causing food poisonings, more so than many foods?

Primarily because poultry has been found to be much more likely than most other foods to be contaminated with food poisoning bacteria, such as *salmonella*, and the relatively new discovery, *campylobacter*. Some estimates are as high as 35-75% or more of raw chicken and turkey that are contaminated with one or both of these bacteria.

There are a few explanations for this hazardous situation. Some experts blame the way poultry is in crowded conditions, others blame the slaughterhouses, still others blame the USDA for tolerating such unsanitary and unhealthy practices, and some even blame the consumers for not following good sanitation practices in the home. Wherever the blame may belong, however, you, as the consumer, should be aware of just how hazardous poultry products may be.

Unfortunately, you can not depend upon sight or smell to detect contaminated chicken or turkey (unless the contamination is so extreme as to cause discoloration and/or a bad odor). This is because in the case of some types of bacteria, such as *salmonella*, it takes only a few bacteria cells to cause serious illness. Your best defense against these bacteria in a restaurant setting, then, is to be quite sure the chicken or turkey you are served is thoroughly cooked and is served either very hot or very cold.

Of all the sources of food poisoning, turkey is the second most common source of salmonella outbreaks due to meat in the U.S. This is because it is usually the hardest to cook all the way through. Beef is the most common source because it often goes through much more processing or handling, such as with hamburger, than other cuts of meat, and this extra processing allows for a greater possibility for contamination. Some experts believe that beef is involved in more reported salmonellosis outbreaks than poultry, even though beef carries much lower levels of *salmonella* bacteria, because so many people like it cooked rare.

There is still the possibility of becoming ill from eating thoroughly cooked poultry or beef if the cooked meat came in contact, either directly or indirectly, with raw or partially cooked meat, which is known as cross-contamination. This can happen very easily if the food handler uses the same utensils, cutting board or table, or even his or her hands for both the raw and cooked meat or other potentially hazardous food without sanitizing in between uses, especially after just handling raw meat.

You can decrease the possibility of becoming ill even if this happens to your food just by assuring that your meal is very, very hot when you receive it. Coldness will not kill harmful germs like heat can. If, though, you have a view into the kitchen area of a restaurant you can then take note of how they handle the raw and cooked potentially hazardous foods. If it looks suspicious don't hesitate to bring it up with the manager and definitely inform the Health Department. I will explain more on cross-contamination and how to prevent it in the section on home food preparation.

EGGS

Some states or localities, because of the following findings, may have enacted, or are possibly in the process of enacting, laws which would require shell eggs to be maintained at refrigeration temperatures.

Since August 1990, the FDA has designated shell eggs as a "potentially hazardous food". This means that retail food establishments must now comply with specific time and temperature controls when handling eggs. The California Health and Safety Code currently lists shell eggs as not being a potentially hazardous food as long as they are not broken or cracked open, and therefore does not require eggs to be refrigerated.

Recent cases of food poisonings have shown that *salmonella* - a common and very dangerous food poisoning bacteria - has been implicated in illnesses and deaths involving whole, disinfected Grade A eggs. *Salmonella* has been associated with food poisonings involving broken or cracked eggs for a long time. New findings have revealed that an undamaged shell egg can become contaminated with *salmonella* from the egg-laying hen, during ovulation, before the egg shell was formed.

The Food and Drug Administration (FDA) and the Centers for Disease Control (CDC) have been strongly advising, since 1988, that consumers "avoid eating raw eggs, and products made with raw eggs such as Caesar salad, homemade eggnog, homemade mayonnaise, Hollandaise sauce, homemade ice cream, béarnaise sauce and other products containing raw or lightly cooked eggs." They stress to "cook eggs thoroughly." Even undercooked, or runny, scrambled and fried eggs have been implicated in some outbreaks, and are not without risk. Risks also increase if eggs or foods containing eggs are held without refrigeration, so refrigeration is recommended as well.

OTHER POTENTIAL HAZARDS

What other types of foods would be considered potentially hazardous? Most soups and salads as well as cooked rice, pasta, fruit and vegetables, as I mentioned earlier. You may not believe raw fruit or vegetable salads to be potentially hazardous, but they can be, once they've been processed and handled.

Every one of us carries on our skin, hair, and in our saliva and nasal discharge, common, normal bacteria which are harmless until given the right environmental conditions (such as food, water, pH level, proper temperature and presence (or absence) of oxygen) to quickly reproduce to large numbers. A sore or cut in your skin produces the right environmental conditions causing the formation of puss - white blood cells - indicating an infection.

Washing your hands thoroughly with soap and water will help eliminate probably most of that bacteria, though it's very possible some will survive or be picked up from different sources after washing the hands (microorganisms are everywhere). Since most restaurant food handlers do not use gloves, we have to assume some of this bacteria will be passed on to the food.

Temperature is the easiest condition to manipulate, in order to kill or inhibit microorganism growth on the food. Control the temperature and you control the harmful bacteria.

FOOD POISONING VS. FOOD SPOILAGE

Perishable foods, as I mentioned earlier, are not always potentially hazardous. All foods which can and eventually will spoil are perishable. Spoilage commonly occurs when microorganisms grow in or on the food to large numbers. Food poisoning microorganisms grow much faster than food spoilage microorganisms. There are other differences and similarities. Food spoilage microorganisms make themselves known to us, through our senses, much more so than food poisoning microorganisms. If the food looks different, smells bad or rotten, or tastes rancid, sour, alcoholic, yeasty, bitter or putrid, there is a better than average chance it is spoiled; meaning the food very possibly has an overgrowth of microorganisms, and this is an obvious sign not to eat it as it can make you sick. The presence of food poisoning microorganisms, however, is not always so obvious.

Food spoilage microorganisms also differ from food poisoning microorganisms in the temperature range in which they are able to reproduce. Most food poisoning microorganisms grow best at temperatures between 50 and 120°F whereas food spoilage microorganisms are able to grow at lower temperatures, such as the refrigerator temperature of 40°F or lower. Food spoilage microorganisms, which are able to grow at these temperatures, include the mold and yeast which grows on such foods as bread and cheese, and the bacteria which eventually spoils milk and other dairy products.

You may remember that I mentioned earlier that bread is not considered potentially hazardous because it does not contain enough water to support rapid growth of microorganisms. Yet, bread, and bakery products in general, are perishable because food spoilage microorganisms can and will grow. Remember that those three conditions apply only to microorganisms which can reproduce relatively quickly and pose an immediate health risk. Food spoilage microorganisms are not such an immediate health risk because they grow slower and are more easily recognized. Many perishable foods should still be kept refrigerated because the cooler temperatures still slow spoilage microorganism growth, thereby increasing the shelf life and maintaining the freshness of the food.

WHAT TO DO

Let's go back now to examining your food once you've received it. What do you think is the best thing to do if you should receive food that is either not at the proper temperature or is spoiled in some way? You should already know at this point that in either case you should not eat it. The question is, should you reorder the same thing or something else altogether? In both cases I would recommend reordering something else altogether, especially in the case of improper temperature.

If you reorder the same thing, the server or cook may either try to reheat or cool down your serving, or the entire batch or stock, and then just either reserve you your original serving or another serving from the same batch or stock. None of these practices, though, are guaranteed to make the food safe again. Once microorganisms have established themselves, by reproducing to large numbers, normal cooking, reheating, or refrigeration will not always make that food safe again, nor is it recommended to try. The safest thing to do is to throw the food out.

The maintenance of foods at either extreme hot or cold temperatures is mainly to inhibit the growth of microorganisms. Thorough cooking does kill most food poisoning microorganisms, but remember there still is a good chance that the food can be recontaminated after being cooked, through handling and cross-contamination. So, whether the food is thoroughly cooked or not, if it is not maintained at the hot or cold temperatures described earlier, microorganisms will be given a chance to reproduce, and, for some species of microorganisms, produce a toxin or poison which can cause illness or death.

This toxin, or poison, will most likely not be destroyed by ordinary cooking or reheating. Again, you're taking a chance in reheating or cooling something that has been out of temperature for possibly two hours or more, which is all it takes. Also, freezing, unlike thorough cooking, in no way kills all microorganisms.

In the case of receiving spoiled food, the server or cook may not like to start over to prepare you the same thing and may just give you another serving from the same batch, or your original serving somehow changed or dressed up with something to make it more appealing. Again, neither of these practices may guarantee that the food will be safe to eat.

Most of us have come across spoiled food in our own refrigerators and we know better than to try and fix it up so it can be eaten. We know, through our senses, that it could be hazardous to eat. Even if the food tastes a little different than normal (this could mean it's hazardous and your senses are only slightly picking it up) don't take the chance. Reorder something altogether different or pick yourself up and go eat somewhere else.

Spoilage can also be caused by other things besides microorganism growth. Frost, heat-drying, excessive humidity can all change the food so as it is no longer appealing in some way. Spoilage in this way and certain spoilage microorganisms, such as those which spoil fruits and vegetables, are not generally harmful to us, though I know most of us would still rather not want to eat these foods. The fact that you may have eaten some spoiled food without any ill effects does not mean that your next encounter will turn out so well.

FOOD POISONING HAZARDS

"WAITER, WHAT IS THAT FLY DOING..."

Another thing I want to mention concerning your food, once it is served to you, is regarding foreign objects in the food. Of course, you should never see any kind of foreign object, including glass, metal, etc. as well as insects, in your food. It can and does happen, though, so just be aware that you should immediately stop eating and notify your server or the management of the problem. I would, again, recommend reordering something different for basically the same reason I stated above, that is, if you still have an appetite. Finding a foreign object in your food is also serious enough that you should notify your local Health Department right away.

Consuming foreign objects is one of a number of different ways of becoming food poisoned other than by microorganisms. I mentioned one possible way earlier when I talked about the importance of separating and proper handing and storage of poisonous chemicals to prevent them from contaminating food. Chemical additives, such as monosodium glutamate (MSG), and sulfites, also can cause illness if used in large quantities or are consumed by people who may unknowingly be allergic to them. Other non microbial food-borne illness occurs from eating poisonous animals or plants. All seafood and mushrooms, for example, must come from an approved (government inspected) source. Non microbial food-borne illnesses are much less common than illnesses caused by microorganisms and can be harder to detect in a restaurant setting, but you should be aware that there are other possible ways of becoming ill, though they occur much less frequently.

Another recommendation, which can very possibly avoid or bypass temperature problems, is to order something which is prepared on the spot. On-the-spot preparation means the meal was not premade hours or days ago and is now sitting under or in a heat lamp, warmer or refrigerator waiting for you to order it. For some types of foods, such as soups and salads (which are commonly blamed for food-borne illnesses), it may not be possible to find a restaurant doing on-the-spot preparation. On the other hand, certain restaurants do on-the-spot preparation for all their foods, and some types of foods are always prepared on-the-spot, and are therefore usually safer. If you're not sure, ask your waiter or waitress.

BEVERAGES

Beverages are not nearly as common a cause of food poisonings as solid foods, at least not in the United States. All of our drinking water is well treated to prevent the spread of water-borne illnesses. Many drinks also contain a natural or added substance, usually acidic, to prevent or slow microorganism growth. Examples of this include soda drinks and many fruit drinks. Alcohol, as well, inhibits microorganism growth.

Just as for solid foods, maintaining beverages at refrigerated or hot temperatures is the easiest, most common way to inhibit microorganism growth. Also, just as for solid foods, certain beverages can spoil. The best example of this is milk. Milk and all dairy products are perishable and potentially hazardous.

DAIRY PRODUCTS

Milk is an interesting drink not only because of the variety of ways we can buy it, but also because of the high degree of regulation it must go through in order to be assured to be safe to drink (more than any other liquid drink). There are two basic types of milk or dairy products that everyone should be aware of when considering transmission of illness: pasteurized and raw milk.

Pasteurization is a special heating and cooling process, of which there are a few different methods. Pasteurization is performed on a number of other foods, besides milk, such as cured meats, fruit juices, bakery goods, eggs, beers and wines. This heating process is just hot enough to kill all the pathogenic (disease causing) microorganisms in the milk or other foods. Other microorganisms can and do survive pasteurization of milk and they are the microorganisms which will eventually spoil the milk or dairy product if it's held past its normal shelf life.

Raw milk, on the other hand, is not pasteurized and is, therefore, more risky. Raw milk has been blamed for illnesses throughout history and still is at present. All raw milk in the United States, though, is certified, which means the cows or goats have been thoroughly checked over by professional people, and are certified to be free of all illness or disease causing organisms. Pasteurized milk products still are generally believed to be safer, although they still are considered potentially hazardous and must, therefore, always remain refrigerated. In any case, dairy products in the U.S. are pretty safe.

SALAD BARS AND BUFFETS

It is fairly common to see a salad bar or buffet-type setting in a restaurant dining area nowadays. A salad bar or buffet setting includes any ready-to-eat food displayed for customer self-service. There are a few important things which are required of self-service bars to safeguard your health. One main requirement is that all openly exposed ready-to-eat food must be shielded so as to block a direct line between the customer's mouth and the food on display. This shield is known as a sneeze guard for the larger displays of food and is usually glass or transparent plastic angled above the food, enough to block possible contamination coming from a customer's mouth (saliva from sneezing, coughing, talking, etc.). If the sneeze guard is not present the exposed food must be covered or shielded by some other method approved by the Health Department.

Other requirements for a salad bar, buffet or other customer self service settings include a utensil with a handle for each food displayed for self service. No one is allowed to touch any of the exposed food with their hands. Also, the proper temperatures must be maintained, as described earlier. The food is usually displayed on ice, or the containers are sitting either in a refrigerated unit or warmer, or the food is sitting under a heating lamp.

PICTORIAL PUZZLE #2

Can you find nine potential health code hazards at this salad bar? Check your answers with my list on page 125.

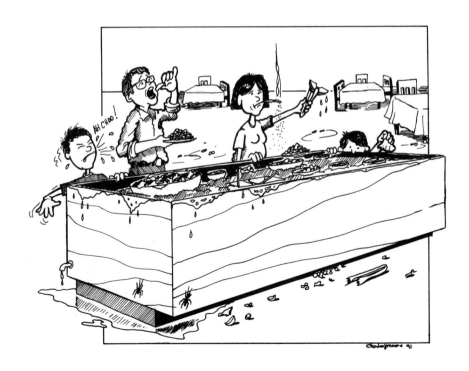

TEMPERATURE MAINTENANCE

Temperature maintenance, especially hot temperatures, is especially important to look out for at self service settings, as well as displayed food, where you pick your food out of a display case and the server puts it on a plate and serves it to you. Temperature is especially important at these settings because very often the food is not being kept hot enough. I have come across many heating lamps which only keep the food warm, not hot, and warming units (or steam tables) which are not turned up high enough to produce any steam. Seeing a heating lamp alone, without a warmer below, is definitely not a good sign and the food under that lamp should just be avoided. For a steam table warmer you should definitely see steam coming up through the food or edges. If you don't, I would recommend avoiding it.

Many hot foods at a buffet may be maintained in a chafing dish, where usually a flame underneath attempts to keep the food hot. I would be suspicious because many times only the food right over the flame is being kept hot enough to be safe and the food towards the corners are only warm. In situations like this the servers should be mixing or stirring the food in the dish so all the food can be kept hot. The servers or staff watching over and maintaining the food also should have and be using probe thermometers on these foods to assure that a minimum temperature of 140°F is being maintained.

For displayed food, which you choose and then a server places on a dish, be careful. If the server takes that food from the warmer and reheats it, perhaps in a microwave, before serving it to you, don't accept this as a safe method. Remember that reheating food, which has been out of proper temperature for an unknown length of time, does not assure it to be safe again. Also, if the server has to reheat it before serving it to you then that almost definitely means the food is not being maintained at the proper hot temperature. The proper legal hot temperature of 140°F or above is hot enough to serve without the food needing to be reheated.

If you come across a buffet setting without proper shield protection or methods of temperature maintenance, which I have seen many times, then chances are the set-up has not been an approved by the Health Department and should be avoided.

Questions like, "How long has the food been sitting at room temperature?" and "Is the food potentially hazardous?" should be considered. Potentially hazardous foods must be maintained at proper temperatures at all times.

SULFITES

Fairly recently laws have been added to the California Health and Safety Codes to protect people who are severely allergic to sulfites. Severe reactions and deaths have occurred from fresheners consisting of sodium or potassium sulfite, bisulfite or metasulfite and sulfur dioxide which were added to foods to maintain their fresh look. This law prohibits the addition of sulfites "to any fruit or vegetable which is sold to be consumed in its raw or natural state" or "any fish or seafood at the wholesale or retail level." Many restaurants were using sulfites on their fruit and vegetables, especially at the salad bar. Sulfites are still being legally used on other fruits and vegetables not sold in the raw state, such as dried fruits, and grapes used for wine. If you suspect a restaurant is possibly using sulfites on their salad bar, don't hesitate to notify your local Health Department. They should investigate it and get back to you on what they found right away.

(e) RESTROOMS

If the kitchen is the most important area of a restaurant when looking for significant violations or hazards to your health, then the toilet facilities or restrooms would probably be a close second. It's therefore always a good idea to check out the restrooms before you eat or order, if only to wash your hands.

People often compare the condition of the restroom to the condition of the kitchen and how the upkeep of the restroom is a good indication of how well the kitchen is being maintained. From my experience as a health inspector I have found that many times this is not always true, especially if the restrooms are well maintained. On the other hand, if the restrooms are not maintained clean and in good overall condition, there is a much better chance that the condition of the kitchen is similar. Remember, also, that there are other things to consider besides cleanliness when evaluating a restaurant's restrooms.

I would always recommend to take a look at the restrooms because, even though they might not reflect the condition of the kitchen, they still can give you a clue as to the sanitary practices of the employees. Some larger restaurants may have separate toilet facilities for employees only, though the majority of restaurants do not. The best way to find out if the customer restrooms are also used by the employees is by observing an employee using them or by simply asking any employee if these are the only restrooms.

CLEAN HANDS

In any case, the restrooms should always have a soap and towel dispenser (or hot air blower). The soap should be a powder or liquid - bar soap is generally not allowed as it has the potential to pass germs from one person to another, and also tends to leave a mess. The soap and towel dispensers should not just be present but also must always be maintained full. If either is missing or empty, especially the soap, take this definitely as not a good sign because chances are the employees are not washing their hands after using the toilet which becomes very hazardous if they handle food.

The microorganisms which can be picked up on the hands of someone, even if they appear healthy, after using the toilet facilities can be very dangerous. The classic example of a food handler who appeared healthy, but in fact was a carrier of *salmonella* and was probably the source of infection for hundreds of people was Typhoid Mary.

"Typhoid Mary" was born Mary Mallon in about 1868 and was first discovered to be a carrier in New York City in 1906. She continued working as a cook, despite orders from health officials, and was repeatedly tracked down through employment agencies that she used. George Soper, a sanitation engineer, connected her to at least 6 typhoid fever outbreaks in New York state. His department documented the cases of at least 53 persons who were infected by Mary Mallon between 1900 and 1915. Three of them died of typhoid fever. She was finally arrested and confined to a hospital for the last 20 years of her life to stop her from continuing to spread the *salmonella* germs.

Typhoid fever is caused by *salmonella typhi*, which is passed through contaminated water or food. Carriers do not have the symptoms of typhoid fever, but they harbor the bacteria in their intestines and release it in their feces. Human wastes containing the bacteria can then contaminate food in several ways.

There still are many people today who are carriers of infectious diseases and aren't aware of it. The normal bacteria found in all of our intestines also can cause us to become ill if given the proper environment and food source to reproduce to large numbers. For these reasons all employees coming in contact with food or food-contact surfaces must wash his or her hands with warm water, soap or cleanser immediately after using the toilet facilities. Legible signs must be posted in all restrooms directing everyone to "wash your hands" after using the toilet to protect the health of yourself and others.

HOT WATER

What else is required of restrooms? Of course, a hand washing sink with both hot and cold running water, and a toilet. Hot water is a must in a food establishment at all hand and utensil wash sinks at all times. If you notice that there is not hot water at the restroom notify your Health Department right away since there is the chance the entire restaurant is operating without hot water.

GENERAL CONDITIONS

The sink, floor, walls and the toilets must always be kept clean and the sink and toilet should never be broken, leaking or backed up. If anything is in disrepair or missing, such as soap or towels, notify the employees or manager and if nothing gets done notify your Health Department, as well.

AVAILABILITY TO CUSTOMERS

One last thing I want to mention concerning restrooms is their availability to the customers. Certain restaurants are not required to provide toilet facilities to their customers, even though most do. It will, most of the time, depend on the size of the food establishment. The larger the establishment, the more likely it is that the law requires them to provide customers access to restrooms. The size requirements may vary from one Health Department to another.

HEALTH DEPARTMENTS

In concluding the subject of restaurants, let me tell you some of the things your local Health Department may be doing to keep the public informed about your local food establishments. One fairly new thing being done in Los Angeles County is providing a listing of the recent closures of restaurants, food markets, etc. and the reasons for closure, (which could be anything from not having a current health permit to vermin infestation, backed up toilet, or no hot water), in the local paper once a month for the public to take note of.

Another thing some Health Departments do is to have a grading system where "A" is excellent and "D" is poor and require the establishment to post that grade in a conspicuous place for the public to see.

Finally, I should mention that some Health Departments, to keep the public informed, require establishments to post in a conspicuous place a copy of their most recent inspection report, listing any violations. Again, this is for the public to see. This one is the most helpful, I believe, for you to evaluate the overall safety of the restaurant or market, because you can easily read just what the violations are and possibly if they've been abated or not, and then decide if you still want to eat there.

Some Health Departments may not require any of these methods or may just be doing something else altogether, which I haven't mentioned here. If you're not sure, check with your Health Department. At present, Los Angeles County Health Department only prints a listing of recent closures in the Los Angeles Times once a month.

FOREIGN COUNTRIES

One last thing I should mention in regards to dining out is the situation in foreign countries. Eating out at a restaurant in another country can really be a whole different experience not only because of the different types of food you will come across but also the different health, sanitation, food handling practices and laws, or lack thereof, you might observe. Like I stated in the introduction, the United States has probably some of the strictest standards for food inspections in the world. This, of course, doesn't mean the rest of the world is unsafe. It merely depends on where you go, even within the same country. (Consult with a travel agent or someone who has been there before you go). Again, though, wherever you go, it can't hurt and I believe can only help, to keep your senses working and use the information described in this book whenever possible.

CATERING TRUCKS

What exactly is a catering truck? Simply put, it is a restaurant kitchen on wheels, or in a more legalistic definition, a mobile food preparation unit. They can cook, handle open food and do other types of food preparation normally only a restaurant could legally do. Do not confuse catering trucks with ice cream and candy trucks or other street vendors which mostly sell only prepackaged foods and very limited types of unpackaged foods. I will discuss these in the next section.

Though a catering truck is not considered a food establishment in the Health and Safety Code, it still must obey most of the same requirements, or laws, as I have just described for a restaurant. To summarize: for food handlers, this includes such things as hair restraints, clean outer garments, good hygiene habits, no tobacco use or expectorating, nor eating while around food. The employees must also be in good health - free of all communicable illnesses.

Other similar requirements include good maintenance and cleaning all equipment, walls, shelves, floors, ceiling, and utensils. The truck must also be free of all vermin and live animals at all times. Food must be stored so as to be protected from all types of contamination, including overhead contamination, chemical contamination, customer saliva (sneezing, coughing) and so on. All food temperature requirements are also the same as a restaurant's. Basically, all the food sanitation requirements are the same as a restaurant's.

One additional thing you can take note of is that a legible name, address and phone number should appear on both sides of the truck. The name can be the owner's, operator's, permittee's business or commissary name. This allows for easy identification by the Health Inspector and the public.

If you ever happen to come across a catering truck that is lacking in many or most of the basic requirements or maybe just doesn't appear to be like most other catering trucks, then there is a good chance that it is not licensed and is operating illegally. The current health permit should be posted in a conspicuous place in or on the truck at all times. If you don't see it, ask the operator to show it to you and take note of the expiration date and other information. If he refuses, take it as a hint not to eat there and notify your Health Department right away. Take down or remember as much information as you can about the truck before calling the Health Department, including the name, address, phone number on the truck, license plate number and location where you observed them selling. You should also report any catering truck to the Health Department, licensed or not, if you become ill from eating something from the truck or if they appear to be violating any of the requirements previously described.

PICTORIAL PUZZLE #3

Can you find six health code violations on this catering truck? Check your answers with the list at the back of the book on page 127.

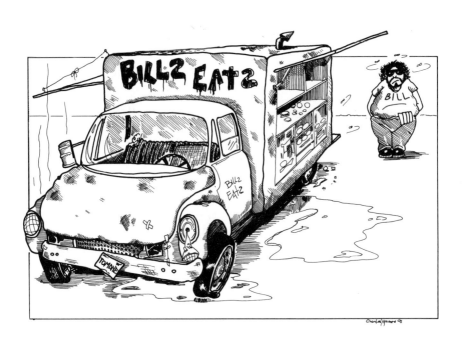

STREET VENDORS

Street vendors, as their name indicates, generally sell their goods to the public on a public street or sidewalk. In the Health and Safety Code, those street vendors which sell any type of food product from a cart or any type of vehicle fall under the definition and section for vehicles, whether they are selling food from a cart, truck (except if it's a catering truck), car or a motorized cart. Whichever they are using it must be approved by the Health Department prior to its use.

LICENSED VEHICLES

There are a number of Health and Safety Code requirements for a vehicle or a street vendor selling food or drinks. I'm going to describe most of the basic requirements here, so that you can very easily distinguish between a legal, licensed vehicle and an illegal one, as far as the Health and Safety Code is concerned.

The chances of getting sick after eating something from an illegal vendor are much, much greater than an inspected, licensed and, therefore, legal one. It is really to everyone's benefit to know the difference, especially since there are so many illegal vehicles out there that have never been inspected and should definitely be reported.

Unfortunately, because street vending has grown tremendously in certain areas over the past 10 to 20 years, some Health Departments haven't been able to keep up with adequate inspections or enforcement on these vendors. It becomes, then, very important that people learn to distinguish a possibly illegal, unhealthful food vendor from a good one and not to patronize the illegal or unhealthful ones for your own protection. Just as for catering trucks, look for or ask to see a current health permit posted in a conspicuous place.

What does the law require of a legal vehicle? First, the law distinguishes between two types of vehicles, depending on whether they sell prepackaged foods, such as candy, ice cream, potato chips, drinks and so on, or foods in the unpackaged state.

Unpackaged foods can only include popcorn, nuts, produce, pretzels, and similar bakery products, candy, hot dogs, snowcones, whole fish and whole shellfish, and hot and cold beverages and only if they are not potentially hazardous and they are sold from an approved bulk dispensing device. Vehicles can sell just about any or all types of prepackaged foods, but they can only sell those unpackaged foods listed above, and nothing else.

REQUIREMENTS FOR ALL VEHICLES

1. All vehicles must have a legible name, address and phone number on both sides of the vehicle just as for catering trucks.

2. All of their equipment and utensils must be sturdy, in good condition and kept clean.

3. Unfinished wood surfaces are not permitted. All of the surfaces, equipment and utensils must be made of nontoxic materials.

4. The food offered for sale cannot be stored, displayed or served from any place other than the vehicle, such as the adjacent ground surface or an extra table.

5. All food condiments must be protected from all types of contamination, such as people sneezing, coughing, as well as bugs, dust or any possible overhead contamination.

6. No food or drinks made or prepared at home or any other unapproved, unlicensed sources, can be sold to the public from any vehicle. (This also applies to all restaurants, catering trucks and food markets).

7. All waste water must drain into an approved water receptor, which also applies to catering trucks. Allowing waste water, of any kind, to drain into the street, gutter, or ground surface is illegal, though a common sight.

8. Proper hot and cold temperatures for potentially hazardous foods must be maintained. Common foods sold from a vehicle which must always be maintained at safe temperatures include hot dogs, fish and other seafood animals, tamales (which can only be sold prepackaged), and ice cream.

9. Vehicle food sales can only be conducted within 200 feet of approved and easily accessible toilet and handwashing facilities - not a home, but a sight approved by the Health Department. (For a catering truck, toilet facilities shall be available within 100 feet of the truck whenever it is stopped to conduct business for more than a one hour period).

10. All food operators must also follow the same requirements regarding good health and hygiene, just as if they were working in a restaurant kitchen.

11. The vehicle must, of course, be free of all vermin and live animals at all times.

ADDITIONAL REQUIREMENTS
FOR VENDORS OF UNPACKAGED FOODS

If the vehicle operator is selling unpackaged foods there are additional requirements for their vehicle than if they were selling only prepackaged foods. One main requirement is a food compartment, completely enclosed on all sides, which may be mainly a plastic or metallic enclosure. This enclosed compartment is required for the sale of any of the unpackaged foods listed earlier, except produce and certain approved beverages, and is mainly for protection of the open food from any possible contamination.

If the vehicle operator is selling unpackaged hot dogs, popcorn or snowcones, there are a few more things the vehicle has to have at all times of operation. The vehicle must have a one-compartment metal sink with a warm (at least 101°F) and cold supply of running water. This sink is used for both washing hands and utensils. Along with the sink there must also be handwashing cleanser and single-service towels (meaning the towels can only be used once and must be discarded or replaced. Paper is preferred). The water supply tank must be of at least 5 gallons, and a waste water tank, as well, of at least 7.5 gallons. Since ice qualifies as a food it must, therefore, come from an approved source (again not from home). Ice will not likely support growth of food poisoning microorganisms but it can still be contaminated in other ways, such as chemical contamination, foreign objects, insects or with other vermin.

For vehicles selling unpackaged whole fish and shellfish the sink, handwashing and water supplies are not required. They are, though, still required to have a waste water tank of at least 7.5 gallons for drainage of waste water (melted ice) from display and storage compartments.

FOOD POISONING HAZARDS

There is one situation where the sink, handwashing supplies, water supply and waste water tank is not required for vehicles which sell unpackaged hot dogs, popcorn, or snowcones and that is if the vehicle operates only on a premises, not the street or any public area, where approved toilet, handwashing and utensil washing facilities are readily available and within 200 feet. This means a private or commercially owned property which allows the vendor to operate on their property, use their facilities and allow the health inspector access to approve and periodically inspect these facilities (again a home would not qualify).

All of these requirements on vehicles or street vendors may sound confusing and hard to remember but they are actually easy to remember once you've visually applied them. If you recall some of the basic requirements such as a name, address and phone number, a posted current health permit in a conspicuous place (which is also a requirement of catering trucks, restaurants and food markets, as well). Try to remember also, that there are two basic types of vehicles depending on whether they sell prepackaged or unpackaged food, and only those unpackaged foods I listed earlier.

BE YOUR OWN HEALTH INSPECTOR

Since you, the customer, can see just about everything on a vehicle or street vendor that a health inspector can (unlike a restaurant or catering truck), you can and should be your own inspector. This is the main reason why I am explaining all of the requirements in such detail.

There are many illegal street vendors out there, especially in areas such as Southern California. The chance of getting sick from an illegal vendor, or even a legal one on which you can see some significant violations, is very high.

One example of a very common illegal vendor is the produce vendor. The fruits or vegetables themselves are mostly safe, though it is mostly stored illegally on the ground or in unapproved, unlicensed containers or vehicles. The produce becomes unsafe when the vendor starts cutting it up and placing it in cartons to sell. Under no circumstances, at least not in California, can a street vendor, licensed or not, cut up or process produce for sale to the public.

Another common illegal, unsafe vendor set-up is the barbecue. I've seen people barbecuing all kinds of meat, corn and more. Most, if not all, of the people operating these illegal, unsafe set-ups have little or no knowledge of how food-borne illness occurs or how to prevent it. It is best for your own health and safety to avoid these and all types of illegal vendors, as well as those legal ones which appear to have significant violations, and to notify your local Health Department when you observe one.

PICTORIAL PUZZLE #4

Can you find eight potential health hazards on this vendor's wagon? Compare your answers with mine at the back of the book on page 128.

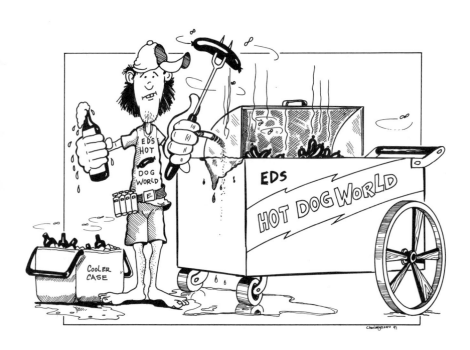

SUMMING UP

In concluding the dining out experience, I should tell you, from mine and other's experiences, that the street vendors are not the only ones out there that lack knowledge of food safety and sanitation. I have met many people, including experienced chefs, cooks and managers, who work at and operate food establishments with years of experience behind them, yet they know very little if anything about safe food handling practices, general sanitation, food-borne illness and the Health and Safety Law, such as I have described in this chapter.

Why this terrible lack of basic knowledge? One likely reason is that many health departments, cities and other local governments and businesses themselves, do not require the manager, food handlers and other employees to know and understand safe food handling practices, general sanitation, food-borne illness or the Health and Safety Laws. This is disturbing not only if you're a health inspector trying to educate these food operators (even when they many times resist being told what they need to do or how they need to do something).

More significantly, this lack of ignorance poses a threat to you the customer who places your health and safety in the hands of those managers and food operators who serve you. Even some of the nicest, most expensive, elegant restaurants I have come across have some ignorant employees. These types of restaurants also get their share of food poisoning complaints.

FOOD POISONING HAZARDS

When it comes to looking after your health you should know that the local health inspector can't be at any one place 100% of the time, or in fact, even a small fraction of the time the establishment is operating, unless a business hires its own health specialists to constantly look over its operation, which is very rare at the retail level. (In California we inspect places about three times a year.)

PROTECT YOURSELF AND YOUR COMMUNITY

You're then left having to trust the management and food handlers or you can use your own senses and common sense, and the tips, clues and laws described in this book to become your own inspector. Also, since the health inspector is only at the restaurant a very small fraction of the time it is operating, you, the customer, should speak up to the employees or management more when you observe a violation or a hazardous situation. I believe the customer can and does make a difference by speaking up, and in many places more so than a health inspector.

Remember, whenever you eat out, the place you choose to eat depends on repeat business to make a profit and stay in business. If you speak up about unhealthful conditions, the management can not afford to ignore these complaints for very long.

Chapter 2

GROCERY SHOPPING

In this chapter I'm going to describe most of the basic requirements, and what to look out for, at both a general food market and at a meat market. Many food markets nowadays have a deli, bakery, meat market or some small food preparation area in addition to the market itself. Since all of these smaller shops or areas do some kind of food preparation or processing, they must follow mostly the same laws or guidelines as a restaurant and what to look out for with respect to those operations has already been covered in the previous chapter on dining out.

FOOD MARKETS

My definition of a food market is any permanently located establishment where food is sold retail in a prepackaged and labeled state to be consumed at another location. Produce is the main exception to this definition in that it can be sold in an unpackaged, unlabeled state. Many markets may also legally have small warmers with anything from popcorn to hot dogs or pizza, all unpackaged and unlabeled. Just be cautious as to proper temperature, handling by employees or other possible contamination of these and other unpackaged, ready-to-eat foods.

A food market has pretty much all of the same requirements as a restaurant. If we start outside, like we did for a restaurant, the trash area and outside grounds must be well maintained. There should be no overflowing, accumulations of trash or any other refuse. Inside the market the employee requirements, maintenance of all equipment, walls, floors, ceiling, shelves; providing a vermin- and live animal-free environment; and proper temperature maintenance of all potentially hazardous foods are all the same as a restaurant. Hair restraints may not be as strictly enforced for employees in a market as in a restaurant, if they only work with prepackaged foods. Dogs used by the blind, signal dogs, service dogs, aquariums and aviaries (properly enclosed) are also allowed, as in a restaurant.

REFRIGERATION

Most food markets have refrigeration and freezer units which allow customer access, unlike a restaurant. All refrigerators in both markets and restaurants, especially if they contain potentially hazardous foods, must not only be maintained clean and in good working order, but must also have a thermometer located inside to indicate the air temperature in the warmest part of the unit and affixed in a readily visible location. In a market then, you, the customer, can check the temperature of just about any refrigerator to be sure that it is maintaining a reading at or below 45°F. Refrigerated food should also feel cold to the touch and frozen food should feel rock solid.

One good tip to remember and practice while shopping at the grocery store is to pick up the perishables as your last stop in the market, especially in hot weather, and always get them home and into the refrigerator right away. Never leave perishable food in a hot car. If you live a good distance away from the store, consider using an ice chest to store the perishables for the trip home.

TOXICS

Another thing to be aware of at a food market is that all poisonous substances, such as detergents, bleaches, other cleaning compounds, insecticides or any other injurious poisonous substance are not stored too close to, and especially not above, food products where they can potentially contaminate that food by leaking or spilling over onto the food.

PACKAGED FOODS

The main thing to be aware of at a food market is, of course, the food itself. You should always take at least a quick look at the packaging of all products you buy to be sure they are well sealed and not torn, damaged, open, spoiled or moldy. If you see a damaged package or spoiled or moldy food, give it to one of the employees to be either disposed of or returned by the store to the manufacturer for credit. Definitely do not buy it. If a food looks any bit suspicious don't buy it. Remember, also, that nothing made or processed at a private home can be sold at a food market (or any other retail food outlet). Every food product sold to the public must come from a government inspected and approved source.

You can usually tell if a packaged food isn't approved by the label or lack of a label. A food package label, in most cases, is required to have at least five pieces of information on it:

1. A common product name.

2. Company or brand name.

3. Address of either producer or distributor.

4. List of ingredients in descending order of amount present.

5. Net weight or volume.

CANNED FOODS

Let me describe now one important type of food packaging - canned foods. Canned foods, whether in tins or glass jars, are of special importance when it comes to avoiding food-borne illness. Canned foods will not keep forever, contrary to what many people may believe. There are limits to how long commercial canning - which is done under tightly controlled conditions - will preserve food. Those limits are affected by rusting, corrosion, and high or low temperatures.

Rusting of cans or lids can occur over time and can cause small holes to open in the can allowing for spoilage to occur. Holes can also be caused by shipping or handling accidents, where cans fall or are crushed or dented. Dented cans , therefore, pose a risk and should not be sold, or their contents consumed, especially if the dent affects the seal on the top or bottom of the can or the seal that runs vertically along the can. You may need to remove the label in order to see the vertical seal.

Corrosion of cans occurs mainly with high-acid foods, like canned tomatoes, where the food continually reacts chemically with the metal container. Over several years this can cause taste and texture changes and eventually lowers the nutritional value of the food.

High temperatures (over 100°F) are also harmful to canned foods by increasing the risk of spoilage. High temperatures can affect the taste, texture and appearance, and also cause increased growth of microorganisms.

Accidental freezing of canned foods left in a car or a basement in sub-freezing temperatures can present health problems. Since water expands when frozen, canned goods can swell and cause the seams to burst or rust in which case the cans should be thrown away. If, though, the cans are only swollen, and you're sure the swelling was caused by freezing, then thoroughly cook the contents right away. You can eat or refreeze the cooked food. If the seams are rusted, though, don't take the chance - just throw the cans out.

Another cause of swelling in canned foods is the growth of microorganisms producing a gas, the most pathogenic of which is the bacteria *clostridium botulinum* - the cause of the deadly food poisoning commonly known as botulism. While botulism is extremely rare in commercially canned foods produced in the United States, it is the worst problem you can encounter in canned foods. The risk is greater if the food is home canned, where there is a greater chance that safe canning procedures have not been followed.

To avoid botulism always examine any canned food, especially home-canned food, before you open it, for possible botulism warnings, such as leaking, bulging, swollen or badly dented cans, cracked jars, or jars with loose or bulging lids, canned food with a foul odor, or any container which spurts liquid when you open it or contains milky liquids, which should

63

be clear, surrounding vegetables. You should not even taste any abnormal canned food, as even a very small amount of botulinum toxin can be very dangerous. Also, it's not recommended to try to open any bulging canned food, since it is under pressure which can cause the contents to splatter. For more details on canned foods see page 105 in Chapter IV., "In Your Own Kitchen".

DRY GOODS

For dry paper or plastic food packages, besides looking for punctures and tears, check to be sure the outside is not damp or moldy. Dampness or mold indicates that the product was contaminated in some way with water or other liquid.

Now, if the product is not damaged or spoiled in some way and is being maintained at the proper temperature, then what else is there to look out for to indicate if the food is safe to buy? There is the "sell by" and "use by" dates printed on many food products, which can be helpful, provided you know how to use them.

PRODUCT DATES

First, the "sell by" date tells mainly the grocer, but also you the consumer, how long the product should be kept for sale on the shelf. The "sell by" date does not mean the product is spoiled and no longer any good after that date, but is more of a recommendation by the producer that the product will start to loose its freshness and quality soon after that date. The grocer is, therefore, recommended to remove the product from the shelf after this date has passed and most likely return it to the producer for credit.

The "use by" date, on the other hand, is intended to mainly let you, the consumer, know how long the product will retain best eating quality after you buy it. Again, this date is a good recommendation by the producer that this product will start to loose its freshness and quality after this date.

Both of these dates are only recommendations, and there isn't a California State Health and Safety Code stating that the seller must remove the product once the "sell by" or "use by" date passes. The Health and Safety Code mentions mainly that it is illegal to keep for sale food which is spoiled, adulterated, or contaminated (in addition to other sanitation requirements), with no mention of product dates. It is, then, a good idea for you to check these dates since the grocer may not, and to bring to his attention any product dates which have passed. Also, because you don't want to be stuck with a food product that may spoil or lose its quality and freshness sooner than you expected, these dates should be used as guidelines for your own purchases. In other words, don't buy anything you won't use before the "use by" date.

Finally, on product dates, you should realize that while these dates are helpful, you can't rely on them absolutely. These dates do not take into consideration a number of things which can shorten a foods useful life, such as too much handling by store employees and customers or improper storage temperature.

MEAT AND SEAFOOD MARKETS

What is it that makes a meat market somewhat different from a restaurant or a general food market? The meat market does both what a restaurant mainly does - food processing - and what a food market mainly does - selling packaged foods to be processed and consumed at another location. This means that a meat market has to abide by all the requirements of both a restaurant and a food market. There are few things you should be especially aware of concerning a meat or seafood market.

A meat market can be defined as any permanently located establishment where both water and land animal parts are processed, displayed, packaged and sold retail, mainly in the raw, not ready-to-eat, state. Some meat markets also have a kitchen where they additionally cook their meat and display it cold or hot for sale ready-to-eat. Whether they cook their meat or not, a meat market must follow all the same requirements as a restaurant and a food market.

There are two basic ways you will see meat or seafood products displayed at a meat or seafood market. One way is prepackaged in a self-service display refrigerator or freezer. The other way is unpackaged in a display case where the butcher or other employee wraps up whatever you point out and request.

PREPACKAGED SELF-SERVICE DISPLAYS

Since meat, poultry and seafood products spoil very easily and quickly compared to other foods, you should always scrutinize the product to be sure it appears to be safe. If it smells bad, or looks discolored, give it to an employee to be disposed of. Discolored meat can look purple or greenish in color, and whitish or bleached for frozen meat, brown for unfrozen lamb, and in pork the darkening of the lean meat and discoloration and the rancid condition of the rind. Spoiled poultry can have soft, flabby flesh, purplish or greenish color, abnormal odor, be sticky under the wings and joints and have darkened wing tips. Spoiled fish can have gray, brown or greenish gills, which feel dry; cloudy, redish, sunken or depressed eyes; soft, easily torn flesh, and a noticeably strong fish odor.

Don't be afraid or embarrassed to smell the fish, even the body cavity. For clams, oysters, mussels the shells should be tightly closed, indicating that they are still alive. If the shell is slightly open tap on it strongly. If it doesn't close, don't buy it.

Check the temperature, also, by feeling the meat, poultry or seafood to be sure it is very cold, and look at the thermometer to be sure the refrigerator is being maintained below 45°F for refrigerators and at 0°F for freezers. Remember that meat products, and especially seafood products, spoil much faster if not maintained at cooler temperatures. If you see meat, poultry or seafood products which appear or smell spoiled notify your local Health Department because the meat market may very likely be doing something wrong in the processing of the meats, causing either unnecessary contamination, or improper storage or processing causing a decrease in their product shelf life.

All meat, poultry and seafood packages sold in a meat market self-service display case will also have a "sell by" date on the label. The "sell by" dates on a meat package are actually, though, less reliable than the "sell by" date on other products. This is because a meat market does much of its own packaging and stamping of "sell buy" dates for many of its products. When the meat product passes that "sell by" date, if the meat, poultry or seafood is not spoiled or contaminated in some way, the meat market can <u>legally</u> repackage the meat, poultry or seafood product with a new "sell by" date. Most meat markets I've come across practice this, which is really all the more reason to examine the meat product before you buy it. In the next chapter, on safe practices in your own kitchen, I've provided a chart listing time limits on different meat and poultry products, after you get them home.

UNPACKAGED CUSTOMER SERVICE DISPLAYS

The other common way to buy meat and seafood products at a meat market is from a display case, where the meat and seafood is displayed, unpackaged. You then request the butcher to wrap up however much you request. This display case can be a completely enclosed refrigeration unit, or an open case with some kind of protection guards, similar to what is required of restaurant buffet settings.

If the display case is a refrigeration unit it must then have a thermometer, though you probably won't be able to see it since it will most likely be facing towards the butcher. You can still check for cold temperature by both feeling the front glass of the display case and your meat package once you receive it, both of which should feel distinctly cold, or ask to see the thermometer.

Besides checking temperature and, of course, observing overall quality for signs of spoilage, you should also look for overhead contamination from the refrigerator apparatus directly above the meat and seafood products. I've come across many of these units which leak water onto the unpackaged, exposed meat and seafood products. This water may just be a buildup of condensation, but even condensation should not come in contact with food and must properly drain out to an approved sewer line or evaporator unit, as it can contain hazardous microorganisms and it did not come from an approved plumbing fixture. Any water, therefore, coming from, or produced by, a refrigeration unit is considered waste water and cannot come in contact with food, or food contact surfaces. This rule applies to all refrigeration units used by restaurants, food markets, catering trucks and street vendors.

If the display case is not a refrigeration unit, then the meat and seafood products will most likely be maintained cold with ice (ice may also be used in a refrigeration unit). Once the ice melts it must drain out of the case to a drain, not a bucket or pan. Meat and seafood products should not be sitting in standing water. New ice will have to be consistently added to the display and water consistently draining out of the display. If the meat or seafood products are being maintained in standing water then you can't be sure that the food is being maintained at the proper cold temperature. Also, as that water starts to warm up to room temperature potentially hazardous and spoilage bacteria start to grow more rapidly and to larger numbers, both on the food and in the water. It's best then to avoid buying any meat or seafood displayed in standing water.

OTHER HAZARDS TO WATCH OUT FOR

Looking now behind or beyond the front display cases, what else can you take note of at a meat market to indicate a possible health hazard? For one thing, since so much handling and processing goes on in a meat market and the employees are working mainly with potentially hazardous foods, both the employee habits and the overall cleanliness of the meat processing areas have to be impeccable. Such things as clean outer garments and cloth towels are very important.

Aprons and cloth towels should not be used for wiping hands. Aprons are mainly to protect the food handlers' clothes from stains and to protect the food from contamination by the food handlers' clothing. Coats and aprons must then be replaced often throughout the day to help control the passing of microorganisms between meat products. Cloth towels should only be used for cleaning and sanitizing cutting boards and equipment and should be used with a sanitizing solution such as bleach and water. Microorganisms, especially bacteria, can very easily grow and rapidly multiply in a moist, dirty or bloody towel or apron. Also, adequate hair restraints should be worn by anyone working in the meat market area.

FLIES

One common hazard you never want to see in a meat market are flies. There are many species of flies which are attracted to animal flesh and blood. A meat market must, therefore, take extra precautionary measures, just as a restaurant should, to prevent flies from entering into the meat market area. One such measure is the proper storage, containment, and frequent pickup of trash products, both inside and outside the market. The meat scraps and cardboard boxes attract flies to the market area, if not handled and stored properly. If you see flies then, in a market, or even in a restaurant for that matter, chances are the employees or operators are incorrectly storing or handling their trash, in addition to probably not practicing good sanitation maintenance of the meat department or kitchen areas.

Some of the things a meat market, or restaurant, might have to help exclude flies, are a strong fan, or air curtain, above the front and back entry ways, and/or self closing entry/exit doors. Seeing these types of things is a good sign, though they will not always be 100% effective in excluding flies.

There are two devices used in meat markets to kill flies once they've already entered the market. One is an automatic insecticide dispenser and the other is an electric fly killer. The presence of these devices indicates that the meat market is having problems excluding the flies, which is not a good sign. As soon as the flies enter into the market they become hazardous. They can very easily contaminate some open food before being killed by electrocution or insecticide, so these devices really can't be counted on too much. Also, the insecticide dispenser and electric fly killer both have restrictions as to where they can be placed in a market, or restaurant, so as to avoid contaminating food. They can't be placed anywhere close to where they can potentially cause overhead contamination of food or food contact surfaces.

The automatic insecticide dispenser is a wall mounted aerosol sprayer which can dispense insecticide spray into a room at preset time intervals. This dispenser cannot be installed directly over, or within a 12 foot horizontal distance, of any exposed, unpackaged food or food contact surfaces, such as cutting boards, meat blocks or any other surface where food is prepackaged and displayed.

The electric fly killer attracts flies with a florescent light, then kills them by electrocution. This device must be maintained at least 3 feet away, in all directions, from any exposed, unpackaged food or food contact surfaces. The electric fly killer should also have easily removable trays, which catch the dead flies, and which must be cleaned at least once per week.

One other fly killing device you might see in a meat market, or restaurant, but which is not approved to be there is, a shell pest strip. They have been known to melt under warmer conditions and contaminate food and other surfaces, so they are too hazardous for areas where open food is stored or processed.

Why is it that flies are dangerous to our health? To explain very briefly: Many species of flies, just as cockroaches and other vermin, are known to carry disease-causing organisms and to have the potential to transmit those organisms to our food. Contamination can occur by just coming into physical contact with the food or food contact surface, or by releasing their saliva onto the food in order to assist in feeding. Contamination also occurs when the body parts of the fly or other vermin somehow become mixed into the food.

FOOD POISONING HAZARDS

Flies and cockroaches, as well as mice and rats, are known for carrying disease causing organisms because for one reason they eat anything and everything, including garbage, fecal matter, raw sewage and so on. Certain species of flies will also deposit live maggots on raw meat very quickly - in just the time it takes to turn away and leave the meat exposed for a few seconds or more. I could go on, but I hope you realize the dangers and will look out and avoid them for your own health and safety and the health and safety of others.

PICTORIAL PUZZLE #5

Okay, one last puzzle for you: There are nine potential health hazards at this meat market. Can you find them all? Compare your answers with my list at the back of the book on page 130.

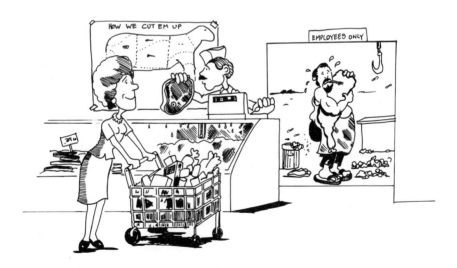

Chapter 3

Fairs, Carnivals, Picnics and Barbecues

> All of these different events have two things in common: They are all temporary events or facilities, and they all serve food that <u>could</u> turn your fun into tragedy. Some require an inspection and public health license, while certain others do not, but the potential for food poisoning is just as real in any of these settings.

In the Health and Safety Code there are two types of temporary food events: temporary food facilities and occasional events. The first, a "Temporary Food Facility", requires a public health license and an inspection in most cases. The second type is called an "Occasional Event", which does not require a public health license, but can still be inspected, although ordinarily only if a complaint is received.

TEMPORARY FOOD FACILITIES

A "Temporary Food Facility" is defined as a retail food outlet operating out of temporary facilities approved by the local Health Department, at a fixed location for a period of time not to exceed 21 days in any 90 day period in conjunction with a single event or celebration, such as a carnival, fair or Christmas sale. Since a temporary food facility serves and sells food to the public, for profit, they are required to be inspected and obtain a Public Health License. Non-profit operations selling to the public may not be required to have a health license or may be exempt from paying the fee for one. Non-profit food stands still, though, must abide by all the Health and Safety Code requirements for a temporary food facility, including the requirement of an inspection.

WHAT TO WATCH OUT FOR

A temporary food facility can be either a restaurant or a food market-type of operation. In most cases, the operator will be doing some type of food preparation, in which case they must follow, for the most part, all the same basic requirements that a restaurant must adhere to.

The booth covering of a temporary food facility must be constructed of either wood, canvas, plastic, tarp or similar material. If there is food preparation going on, most if not all sides of the booth will have to be completely enclosed using fine mesh fly screen or other approved material. One side or window may be allowed to be open depending on whether flies, insects or other possible means of contaminating the food are present. Everything possible must be done to minimize the entrance of insects. If only prepackaged foods or beverages are sold, then fly screening is not necessary.

Also, take note of the condition of the floor. Dirt or earth floors are not allowed. Such floors should be covered with materials such as clean canvas, wood or cleanable carpeting. The use of sawdust or similar materials on the floor is also not permitted.

All food sold from a temporary food facility must be prepared either in an approved, licensed food establishment, or on the premises of the temporary food facility. No food or beverage stored or prepared in a private home can be offered for sale, sold or given away from a temporary food facility, with the exception of non-perishable home prepared bakery products which can be sold from non-profit food stands only.

The proof of purchase invoices should be kept on site so that the inspector or yourself can check to see that the food was not prepared in an unlicensed facility. If you're suspicious or unsure of the food's origin then don't risk your health. Remember that foods produced, especially when mass produced, in a home or other unlicensed facility, are more likely to cause illness, injury or death, than foods produced in a licensed facility.

FOOD PREPARATION

Concerning food preparation, storage protection, temperature, employee habits, equipment condition and vermin, a temporary food facility has to follow the same requirements as a restaurant or food market. All food, including ice and beverages, must be protected at all times from any sort of contamination, and all potentially hazardous food must be maintained at proper temperatures at all times.

Other things required of a temporary food facility include the use of single service utensils only. The operators can only provide their customers with utensils, cups, and plates which are thrown away after you're finished. Also, you should be aware that all customer self-service of unwrapped or unpackaged foods is generally prohibited, meaning a salad bar or buffet-type setting, where you help yourself, is not allowed.

There may be food set out on display but it can only be dispensed by the operators and should be protected, using either sneeze guards or covers, from customer contamination and other forms of contamination.

An open flame barbecue is not too uncommon a site at fairs and carnivals. The barbecue, though, must be located adjacent to the food stand, but not in an area which would allow for customer or overhead contamination.

Live animals, birds or fowl are not permitted in any temporary food facility. The food stands or booths can not be located within 35 feet of animal petting or storage areas, nor positioned under trees or vegetation.

You should also be aware that any waste water produced from the food facility operation must be drained or disposed of legally - meaning down an approved sewer drain line. The operators can not have any kind of drain water or other types of waste water, which includes melted ice, running onto the ground surface where children or animals can come in contact with it.

FOOD SERVERS

What about toilet and handwashing facilities? Of course toilet facilities, at least one toilet for every 15 employees, must be provided within 200 feet of the food stands; and handwashing facilities must be provided in a permanent building or vehicle, within 100 feet of the food stands, with hot and cold running water and liquid or powdered soap and paper towels.

Lastly, remember that smoking, or other tobacco use, and expectorating by employees is not allowed in any temporary food facility. The employees preparing and/or handling food must wear hair restraints, clean outer garments, maintain their hands clean and free of all sores, or cuts and the employees must be in good health - free of all potentially communicable illnesses. Also, children can legally work in a temporary food facility as long as they are working under the direct supervision of a responsible adult.

OCCASIONAL EVENTS

An "occasional event" is an event which occurs not more than three days in any 90-day period, or an average of once per month and does not primarily serve the general public. This type of event includes such things as a church or private club event, or other non-profit association or private gathering where food is sold or given away only to its members or guests. Many private clubs have permanent restaurants or snack shops. Even though they serve only to their members and not to the general public, they are not considered a temporary or occasional event. They are required to abide by all of the rules and regulations that apply to a public restaurant or market.

Most Health Departments will probably not inspect these types of events, unless a complaint is received because these events do not serve the general public. There are usually no Health and Safety Laws which cover food sanitation, employee habits, structures and so on that are legally binding for an occasional event.

An occasional event can, therefore, be one of the most potentially hazardous situations you might come across. Also, bear in mind that, as stated in the introduction to this book, most cases of food poisoning are due to improper food handling or storage in the home, and at many occasional events you might attend there will probably be some food, if not most of the food, prepared at private homes.

HOW TO KEEP YOUR EVENT HAPPY AND HEALTHY

Even though an occasional event may have all these strikes against it, it can still be a safe and happy experience with use of a little knowledge and common sense. I hope I've already passed on some knowledge, clues and tips that will help you protect yourself from food-borne illness at most retail food outlets. Now I'm going to describe some clues and tips to bear in mind with regards to private events.

To start, I would remind you to always try to keep in mind the general kinds of foods which are or are not considered potentially hazardous (though most foods at an occasional event would probably be classified as potentially hazardous). Again, also be cautious of the food's present temperature and past temperature maintenance. If the food has been left out at room temperature or is only being maintained warm and not hot, then a fair rule to follow is to be sure that period of time does not exceed 2 hours. It may be hard to assure this time period, but if you can't, then it's best to avoid that particular food altogether.

SALADS

Salads, including chicken, egg, meat, seafood, potato, pasta and so on, are common at occasional-type of events and are also common sources of food poisoning bacteria. Salads are generally more dangerous than many other types of food at an occasional event, not only because they may contain potentially hazardous food, but also because of the greater amount of processing and preparation which goes into them. This leads to the greater possibility of introducing food poisoning microorganisms or other contaminants. There is also a good possibility that they will not be properly refrigerated all the time, but sitting for long periods of time on display, at room temperature.

I'm not saying that you should never again eat salads at an occasional event, only to be cautious. Take into consideration external factors, such as temperature, appearance and even the taste of the food, as well as who prepared it, and if you're at all familiar with this person's food handling and sanitation practices as well as their health and appearance - no cuts or sores, especially on their hands. Also consider if you've ever eaten food prepared by them before. All these factors and more, as I will describe, considered together can give an overall picture of the food's safety.

One basic mistake made in preparation of salads occurs whenever the meat, chicken or seafood part of the salad is prepared and cooked first. While the meat is cooking, the cook will prepare the rest of the salad and mistakenly, or unknowingly, use the same utensils, dishes, cutting board, etc., used in preparing the meat part of the salad, without sanitizing them with hot water and soap or some kind of sanitizing solution or washing their hands after finishing with the raw meat and starting to work on the other ingredients for the salad.

Microorganisms which were on the raw meat, poultry or seafood can be passed to the remaining salad parts from the unsanitized, unwashed utensils or hands.

Another thing to be cautious of, especially in salads, is undercooked meat, poultry, seafood products or eggs. Raw or undercooked meat and egg products can be more dangerous in a salad because there is more food available for microorganism which survived the undercooking, as well as friendlier temperatures to assist in that growth. It's always a good rule of health, as I mentioned earlier, to eat only thoroughly cooked meat, poultry, eggs and seafood products.

HEALTH FOR THE ASKING

We're all bound to come across certain dishes at an occasional event which we're unfamiliar with and probably have never eaten before. It's always a good idea then to ask what it contains before trying it. You not only get an idea of how potentially hazardous it might be, but also if it contains something you might be allergic to.

Speaking of allergies, remember that sulfite products are prohibited from being used on salads at restaurants, but may still be used by someone at an occasional event to make their fruit, vegetables or other products appear more fresh. Be very cautious then, if you are allergic to sulfur.

THE "CAFETERIA BUG"

Something else to look out for at occasional events are large, deep pots, bowls or containers of thick soups, stews, beans, etc. with a height of approximately 6-8 inches or more. These types of foods in deep containers can take very long to cool down, especially towards the middle of the container. Depending on the size, they can sometimes take a full day <u>or more</u> to cool down to 45°F or below, and that is while being maintained in a good refrigerator. This means that the food was out of temperature for far more than enough time to allow microorganisms to reproduce themselves to large numbers and produce possibly poisonous by-products.

The bacteria commonly associated with this type of food poisoning is called *clostridium perfrigens*, also called the "cafeteria germ" or "bug" since cafeterias commonly use large pots and containers. This bacteria can survive cooking temperatures which would kill other bacteria by forming a very temperature resistant spore cell. These spores are tricky because at temperatures between 70° and 120° F they become normal reproductive cells again and produce a poison which can make you sick. The spores of this bacteria, just like those of botulism bacteria, are everywhere in the environment - in the soil, in the intestines of animals, and in all food. It should be assumed for your own safety's sake that any food you eat is potentially contaminated with them to some extent.

The spores themselves are not hazardous. It is only when the spores change into reproductive cells that they pose a threat to your health. This bacteria's spores (like *clostridium botulinum* - botulism bacteria) can, though, only become reproductive cells at those temperatures just mentioned and only in an environment with little or no oxygen, such as in thick soups, stews, beans, and in canned or bottled food not properly preserved.

Botulinum and *perfrigens* are very much alike, although botulism as a disease is much less common and usually occurs in connection with improper canning techniques. Still, cases have been documented in which cooked foods were the source of botulism.

These types of foods, and others which thicken upon cooling, should be distributed to shallower containers no longer than 30 minutes after the heat is turned off, in order to cool faster and more efficiently. My recommendation then, at an occasional event, is to avoid those thick, soupy foods possibly prepared and/or stored and served in large, deep containers. I would also recommend keeping this practice in mind when preparing large quantities of these types of foods at home, and to always be sure to keep them hot or cold enough to prevent any bacteria from reproducing. Transfer these thick foods to shallow pans for quick cooling in the refrigerator.

BARBECUES

Barbecuing meats, especially chicken, can be more hazardous than normal cooking for a number of reasons. It is common to mistakenly undercook the meat, since a barbecue is usually not as efficient in producing heat and cooking evenly as compared to a stove or oven. Another common error around the barbecue is use of the same utensils, plates or platters for both the raw and cooked meat, allowing cross-contamination to occur. A similar problem arises when marinades are used, in which first the raw meat has been soaked, and then the same marinade is basted onto the meat during the final moments of cooking. You should be aware of these potential hazards at your own barbecue, as well as temporary events you may attend or participate in.

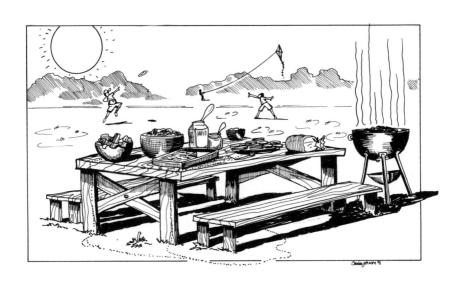

FOOD POISONING HAZARDS

THE CHOICE IS YOURS

Another fairly good tip is that if you have a choice between foods prepared at someone's home or other unlicensed facility, and foods prepared at a known licensed restaurant then I would recommend choosing, diplomatically of course, the food prepared at the licensed establishment. Even though there are a lot of ignorant food handlers working in restaurants these days, I would still tend to believe that the general public probably knows even less than these food handlers. Again, you should take into consideration who prepared the homemade meal and if they appear to know and be following food safety and sanitation practices. You should also take into account the history of the particular type of dish and if you're familiar with its likelihood to cause illness.

PROTECT YOURSELF AND OTHERS

Lastly, I would suggest, when attending an occasional event, to take note of the whole setup, including its operation and surroundings - whether you're inside or out - and recall what would be required if this were a licensed, inspected facility. Remembering and predicting possible ways, or routes, of contamination of the food, or food contact surfaces, will help in determining the safety of any situation where food is handled and managed. The problem with people, both working with the food and eating it, is mainly in knowing what could be a potential or possible contamination or hazard. I hope this book has shed some light on this subject, so you can better judge each situation you find yourself in.

If an occasional event occurs regularly and they serve to a fairly large group of people, then you can make a complaint to your Health Department if you observe some hazardous situation going on. An inspector should investigate your complaint and will probably, if anything, give recommendations to eliminate any hazardous situations.

Since it is not a licensed facility that serves to the general public, the health inspector will probably not be able to issue orders for compliance. If someone, or yourself, does become ill, though, from eating at an occasional event, the Health Department should definitely be notified in the same manner as if it was a licensed facility, so they can investigate, and try to determine the cause in order to prevent it from occurring at similar future events. In most cases, the people operating the food stand event will clean up their act without the need for any legal action, since ignorance is usually the real problem and no one wants to spread disease to others intentionally. A little friendly advice can prevent a lot of disease in cases like this.

Chapter 4

In Your Own Kitchen

> What else is there to know about avoiding food-borne illness? Plenty. The fact that this is the last situation covered in this book does not in any way imply that it is the least important or least likely place to encounter food poisoning. On the contrary, your own kitchen is, in fact, probably the most important, especially for those of us who prepare and eat most of our meals at home.

Your own kitchen is the one place where you have the most control over your own health and the health of others you prepare meals for. It is therefore your responsibility to make sure you prepare and store foods and utensils in a safe and sanitary manner.

In addition to food sanitation, and Health and Safety Laws and practices I've covered so far in this book, there are still a number of specific things you should consider and practice when preparing, handling and storing foods and utensils in your own kitchen. All of these practices I'm about to describe are very good recommendations to follow (primarily based on findings of the U.S. Department of Agriculture) to prevent food-borne illness and the spread of infection.

FOOD POISONING HAZARDS

KEEP IT CLEAN

To start, keep all your washing and drying cloths clean and throw out dirty or mildewed sponges. Bacteria and other germs can survive for periods of time in towels and cloths, especially if they are damp, and can be continuously passed to food or food contact surfaces. Putting your frequently used, damp sponge in the microwave for about 30 seconds or so, until it's steaming, will destroy most, if not all, microorganisms, which is one of the main goals in food preparation safety. It is also a good practice to simply replace sponges every few weeks.

Always wash with hot soapy water or a sanitizer - a solution of water and either chlorine or iodine. Wash your hands, countertops, utensils, etc., between each step in food preparation. I've already mentioned this practice when preparing salads containing meat, poultry, seafood, or eggs, but you should actually perform this practice when working with any of these or other potentially hazardous foods. Bacteria and other microorganisms from potentially hazardous foods can get into or onto other foods, directly or indirectly, if you're not careful to wash everything they've touched before exposing another food to the same surface or utensil.

AVOID CROSS CONTAMINATION

This also means to wash everything between contact with raw meats, poultry, seafood, eggs and other potentially hazardous foods in their raw, uncooked, state and the same food after it has been cooked. It may have been a common practice for you to use the same dish or utensils when marinating or preparing a meat dish both before and after cooking. It is actually much safer and easier, though, to just grab another plate or utensil, since you should always thoroughly wash that used plate or utensil with hot soapy water before using it again.

THE CUTTING BOARD

There may be other places in your kitchen where bacteria can hide, or where you can't reach them with normal cleaning. In certain places, like your cutting board, bacteria can contaminate your food the instant it comes in contact with the surface of the cutting board. The small cracks and crevices which develop in every wood cutting board from knife marks, drying or aging can harbor many germs. *Salmonella* bacteria, which take very few cells to cause serious illness, is just one of the types of bacteria which typically hide in such places as your cutting board's cracks and crevices.

Thousands of bacteria can survive for long periods in a single knife mark, and wiping down the cutting board with hot soapy water will not always remove them.

If you have uncleanable cracks and crevices in your cutting board you have only three alternatives:

1.) You can use a sanitizer, such as chlorine bleach and water (about 1/4 cup bleach per gallon of water) after every use of the cutting board with potentially hazardous foods;

2.) You can fill in all the cracks and crevices with some kind of hardening filler, (which may not be very safe to use, as it may chip and get into the food itself over the course of time); Or,

3.) You can throw out the old cutting board for a new acrylic board which won't develop cracks so easily.

A similar problem exists in the case of wooden handles on knives and should be dealt with in a similar manner.

FOOD POISONING HAZARDS

PERSONAL HYGIENE

There are a few things you can do to prevent the spread of infection or contamination of food from yourself to others:
1. If you're sick, don't handle or prepare food for anyone else.

2. Try not to sneeze or cough anywhere in the kitchen area whether you're sick or not.

3. Wash your hands in hot, soapy water before beginning food preparation and wear gloves when handling food if you have any kind of skin cut or infection on your hands.

4. Maintain a dispenser of liquid or powdered sanitary or antiseptic, antimicrobial soap at your kitchen sink for convenience, and use it often.

ORGANIZING A HEALTHIER HOME

There are also some things to consider when you look around the kitchen and the rest of your home:

1. Prevent contaminants from getting into your food by keeping pets, household cleaners and other chemicals away from food.

2. Don't store food near or below chemicals and leaking pipes.

3. Control vermin by keeping all surfaces clean and sealing all holes or other hiding places in your kitchen and home.

4. If you need to remove any chemical or dry food from its original package or container, take a marking pen and write on the container itself, in large letters, exactly what's being stored in it. It may be obvious to you, but someone else may take and

possibly use that chemical as a food product. (Restaurants are actually required to mark all unlabeled containers to prevent an employee from possibly using the wrong product.)

When working with raw meats, poultry, and seafood you should always assume that they could be contaminated with microorganisms which can cause illness or death. I already described how you should wash every utensil which comes in contact with these foods, but also be careful not to allow raw meat juices to drip onto other foods or utensils. If you wash meat or poultry under cold water before cooking (which is a good idea) be sure afterwards to rinse or wash your sink with hot soapy water. Remove any plates or other utensils from the sink before washing the meat.

Also, be careful of where you store potentially hazardous foods in the refrigerator. Meat juices can leak onto other foods stored just below. It is a good idea to place packages of raw meat, poultry or fish on a plate.

To assure that food is thoroughly cooked all the way through, especially for large birds, consider using a probe-type thermometer to measure its temperature. Instead of cutting into the food to see if it's done, a probe thermometer can give you an accurate reading to see if it's cooked through. To get the most accurate temperature reading the temperature sensitive part of the probe thermometer must be inserted into the thickest part of the meat or poultry (into the thigh), avoiding fat or bone.

USDA RECOMMENDED MINIMUM COOKING TEMPERATURES

The U.S. Department of Agriculture recommends the following minimum temperatures meats should be cooked (throughout the piece of meat) to kill food poisoning organisms:

Ground Meat & Meat Mixtures
Veal, beef, lamb, pork	no less than 160°F
Turkey, chicken	no less than 170°F

Fresh Beef
Medium	no less than 160°F
Well Done	no less than 170°F
Hamburger	no less than 170°F

Fresh Veal
Medium	no less than 160°F
Well Done	no less than 170°F

Fresh Lamb
Medium	no less than 160°F
Well Done	no less than 170°F

Fresh Pork
Medium	no less than 160°F
Well Done	no less than 170°F

Ham
Pre-cooked (to reheat)	no less than 140°F
Fresh (raw)	no less than 160°F

Poultry
    Chicken   **no less than 180-185°F**
    Turkey   **no less than 180-185°F**
    Boneless Turkey Roasts   **no less than 170-175°F**
    Stuffing (inside or
    outside the bird)   **no less than 165°F**

Eggs & Egg Dishes
    Eggs   **Cook until yolk white & firm**
    Egg dishes   **no less than 160°F**

Cured Pork
    Ham, raw   **no less than 170°F**
    (cook before eating)
    Ham, fully cooked   **no less than 140°F**
    (heat before serving)
    Shoulder   **no less than 170°F**
    (cook before eating)

Game
    Deer   **no less than 160-170°F**
    Rabbit   **no less than 180-185°F**
    Duck   **no less than 180-185°F**
    Goose   **no less than 180-185°F**

Note that I didn't mention rare beef because some food poisoning microorganisms may survive, and so it is <u>never</u> recommended.

Also ham, even though it's cured - and often smoked, aged and dried - can still spread food poisoning bacteria and should be handled like any other potentially hazardous food. Always read the label before serving the ham. "Fully cooked" hams have been completely cooked during processing and so they can be served hot or cold. If not precooked, where the label may read "cook before eating", you must, yourself, cook the ham completely through to a uniform internal temperature of 160°F, just as for fresh pork.

COOKING TIPS

Here are some other cooking tips for a safe meal:

1. For cooking frozen food, generally allow 1-1/2 times the period of time required for food that has been thawed. For example, if fresh, unfrozen takes 1/2 hour, allow frozen 3/4 hour.

2. Always cook meat, poultry and other potentially hazardous foods completely through in one cooking. Partial cooking can cause bacterial growth before cooking is complete. Also, some bacteria may survive partial cooking as in hamburger that is red in the middle, rare and medium steaks and roast beef.

3. Cover leftovers and use the probe thermometer to reheat food and make sure it's heated all the way through. The minimum temperature, for reheating foods, should reach at least 165°F. Bring sauces, soups and gravies to a boil. Remember that just because it doesn't taste bad doesn't mean it's completely safe, so heat all leftovers completely through.

4. To check visually, red meat is done when it's brown or grey inside, poultry juices run clear and fish will flake with a fork.

5. Cook eggs until the yolk and white are firm, not runny. Scramble eggs to a firm texture.

6. Never leave food out for more than two hours. Try to leave food at room temperature for as little time as possible. Cooling just cooked, hot food at room temperature can be a dangerous practice, especially if you're not aware or forget how long it stays out. Besides, the notion that food is going to spoil if you put it in the refrigerator soon after cooking it while it's still hot is a myth. Spoilage will more readily occur if the food is held out at room temperature where microorganisms grow best. In fact, placing food in the refrigerator soon after cooking it will

bring it down to a safer temperature more quickly, thereby preventing microorganisms from having enough time to grow. This is safer than leaving cooked foods out at room temperature. Better restaurants often place a container of hot food into a sink full of ice in order to cool it down quickly and safely before refrigerating.

7. Divide large portions of food into small, shallow pans or containers spread out in the refrigerator, not stacked on one another, to allow for more rapid cooling. Remember that large, deep containers of thick sauces, soups, stews, beans, etc. can take hours or even a full day to cool down.

MICROWAVE COOKING

Another type of cooking, which takes special precautions, is microwave cooking. Microwaves are extra-short radio waves that are generated inside the oven and cook food by causing movement (friction) inside the food. Cooking begins just below the food's surface, and spreads through the rest of the food.

Though microwave cooking is quick, it doesn't always cook the food evenly. You may either have to rotate the food or try using the middle temperature range settings. Slower cooking at lower temperatures ensures more even cooking. Also, many microwave recipes may call for a 10 to 15 minute standing time following cooking to allow the heat to spread evenly throughout the food.

It's recommended to always remove large bones from meat before microwave cooking, since bone can act as a shield for the meat surrounding it, thereby preventing thorough cooking. Again, use your probe thermometer and check several spots in the food.

FOOD POISONING HAZARDS

Lastly, for microwaves, do not use the microwave for home canning or heating of any closed containers. Pressure can build up inside the container causing it to explode.

REFRIGERATION TIPS

1. Leave products in their store wrap unless it's torn, in which case rewrap the product in wax paper, plastic wrap, sealable plastic bags, or aluminum foil.

2. Read the labels on all canned meat and poultry products and refrigerate if necessary. All other cans should be kept in a cool, dark place.

3. To avoid freezer burn (which appears as white, dried out patches on the surface of meat) wrap freezer items in heavy freezer paper, plastic wrap, a sealed bag, or aluminum foil. Though freezer burn won't make you sick, it does make meat tough and tasteless.

4. If you have a large supply of frozen foods, you should rotate new items to the back and old items to the front of the freezer. Dating freezer packages, if not already dated, with the date you purchased it, is also a good idea when storing a large supply of food for long periods of time.

5. The safest way to defrost potentially hazardous foods is to take the food out of the freezer and leave it overnight in the refrigerator, never on the kitchen counter at room temperature. Bacteria can grow in the outer layers of the food before the inside thaws.

6. If you need it defrosted sooner, the safest ways include either cooking the food, or using the microwave to either cook or defrost the food, or placing the frozen package in a watertight

plastic bag, if not already in one, under cold water, changing the water often. The cold water temperature will slow bacterial growth. Defrosting foods by leaving them at room temperature is a dangerous practice and is never recommended.

7. Freeze fresh meat, poultry or fish immediately if you can't use it within two to three days.

8. Since the "sell by" dates, printed on meat, poultry and seafood products, are not always very accurate in determining the meat's freshness, it is recommended not to store these products in the refrigerator unless you plan on using it in a day or two. They can be stored much longer in a freezer. (See cold storage chart on the next page).

9. You should have in your refrigerator and freezer easily readable thermometers, placed in the warmest part of each compartment, so you can check to be sure the refrigerator is being maintained at 40-45°F and your freezer at 0 °F or colder.

10. Pack lunches in insulated carriers with a cold pack and carry picnic food in a cooler with a cold pack. Caution children to never leave lunches in direct sun or on a warm radiator.

11. Keep cold party food on ice or serve it throughout the gathering from platters stored in the refrigerator until they are needed.

The chart on the following pages gives conservative cold storage times, as recommended by the U.S. Department of Agriculture, which will help protect yourself from food spoilage (which happens with long refrigeration) and from taste loss (which happens with long freezer storage time).

USDA RECOMMENDED
COLD STORAGE TIMES

Product	Refrigerator Days at 40° F	Freezer Months at 0° F
Fresh Meats		
Roasts (Beef)	3 to 5	6 to 12
Roasts (Lamb)	3 to 5	6 to 9
Roasts (Pork, Veal)	3 to 5	4 to 8
Steaks (Beef)	3 to 5	6 to 12
Chops (Lamb)	3 to 5	6 to 9
Chops (Pork)	3 to 5	3 to 4
Hamburger, ground and stewed meats	1 to 2	3 to 4
Variety Meats (tongue, brain, kidneys, liver and heart)	1 to 2	3 to 4
Sausage (Pork)	1 to 2	1 to 2
Cooked Meats		
Cooked meat and meat dishes	3 to 4	2 to 3
Gravy and meat broth	1 to 2	2 to 3

Processed Meats (Frozen, cured meat loses quality rapidly and should be used as soon as possible.)

Bacon	7	1
Frankfurters	7*	1 to 2
Ham (whole)	7	1 to 2
Ham (half)	3 to 5	1 to 2
Ham (slices)	3 to 4	1 to 2
Luncheon Meats	3 to 5*	1 to 2
Sausage (smoked)	7	1 to 2
Sausage (dry, semi-dry)	14 to 21	1 to 2

USDA RECOMMENDED
COLD STORAGE TIMES
(Continued)

Product	Refrigerator Days at 40° F	Freezer Months at 0° F
Fresh Poultry		
Chicken and		
turkey (whole)	1 to 2	12
Chicken pieces	1 to 2	9
Turkey pieces	1 to 2	6
Duck and		
goose (whole)	1 to 2	6
Giblets	1 to 2	3 to 4
Cooked Poultry		
Covered with broth, gravy	1 to 2	6
Pieces not in broth or gravy	3 to 4	1
Cooked poultry dishes	3 to 4	4 to 6
Fried chicken	3 to 4	4
Game		
Deer	3 to 5	6 to 12
Rabbit	1 to 2	12
Duck and goose (whole, wild)	1 to 2	6

*Once a vacuum-sealed package is opened. Unopened vacuum-sealed packages can be stored in the refrigerator for 2 weeks.

99

MOLD

Unlike bacteria, molds can grow under harsh conditions which would not support other microorganisms. Conditions such as cold refrigeration temperatures, high salt or sugar content, with little moisture, are enough to support these airborne spores which are everywhere.

Molds hasten food spoilage and cause allergic and respiratory problems. A few molds produce mycotoxins or poisons. Both the USDA and the Food and Drug Administration ensure that foods at high risk for toxic mold growth are safe when they arrive at your grocery store. It's up to you to handle any mold growth that occurs after you get foods home. Problems with molds usually occur in the refrigerator.

Most molds look white for the first few days of active growth. When you see a blue, green, grayish or whatever color spot on some food that's an indication that the mold has been growing for two to three days by now and has already begun producing spores that have spread out to the other foods in your refrigerator.

The surface of the mold growth is really only the tip of the iceberg. The larger part of the plant is made up of root threads below the surface. This is where the poisons are contained in those molds which produce mycotoxins.

If you come across mold in your refrigerator you should definitely not sniff or smell the moldy food. You should avoid inhaling any spores which could cause respiratory problems. If the food is heavily covered with mold, wrap it in plastic wrap or a paper bag to keep the spores from infecting the rest of the room. Clean the refrigerator and examine other foods. Mold spreads quickly among fruits and vegetables.

If the food shows only a spot of mold use the following rules of thumb:

Cheese:

For those hard cheeses that are not supposed to have any mold (some cheese is actually made from beneficial molds) cut off at least an inch around and below the spot of mold. Don't touch the spot with your knife or cheese wire. After removing the mold, re-wrap the cheese in fresh plastic wrap. Don't try to save individual cheese slices, soft cheese, cottage cheese, cream, sour cream, or yogurt.

Hard salamis & Dry-cured country hams:

Follow the cheese rule, and keep the knife out of the mold. Don't save moldy bacon, hot dogs, sliced lunch meats, meat pies or opened canned hams.

Smoked Turkey:

Cut a small spot, again using the cheese rule. Throw out moldy baked chicken.

FOOD POISONING HAZARDS

Jams & Jellies:

A tiny spot can be safely scooped out. Then get a second clean spoon and scoop out a large amount of the jam or jelly closest to the spot. If the remainder looks and smells normal, then you can use it. If it tastes fermented, throw it out.

Fruits & Vegetables:

You can cut away small spots of mold from the surface of firm fruits and vegetables, such as cabbages, bell peppers or carrots, but discard any soft vegetables such as tomatoes, cucumbers or lettuce, that show mold growth.

Throw Away On Sight:

Visibly moldy bread, cakes, buns, pastry, corn on the cob, stored nuts, flour, whole grains, rice, dried peas or beans, and peanut butter. Pay special attention to health foods or "natural" foods which are processed without preservatives. They are at high risk for mold growth.

To prevent mold from spoiling your food you have to protect it from the spores. Keep it covered using plastic wrap or at least paper towels and don't leave perishables out of the refrigerator for more than two hours. Mold can grow well in the refrigerator and then even faster at warmer room temperatures. Finally, refrigerate canned and vacuum-packed items after opening. Air which gets in after the seal is broken can promote mold growth.

POTENTIALLY HAZARDOUS FOODS

There are a number of specially prepared, potentially hazardous foods which require extra precautions because they are particularly vulnerable to food poisoning bacteria. A common example is poultry with stuffing.

The starchy dressing of stuffing can readily support bacterial growth - introduced into the stuffing from contact with the raw poultry. To avoid giving any bacteria from the raw poultry a chance to grow in the stuffing, you should mix your stuffing a day ahead of time, premixing only the dry ingredients, and refrigerate it separately from the uncooked bird. Also, keep the stuffing separate from the bird until you are ready to cook it, and then stuff it loosely, which will allow the heat from the oven to cook the stuffing all the way through. Use a probe thermometer to be sure the temperature of the stuffing reaches 165°F all the way through and that the temperature of the bird reaches 185°F, to be fully cooked. Leave the thermometer in place for a minute or so, for an accurate reading.

When it's ready to serve, place the stuffing in a separate container for serving and refrigeration of leftovers.

For commercially frozen stuffed poultry, such as rock cornish hen, you should never thaw such food products before cooking. Follow the directions carefully on the storage and cooking of such items.

Another very common, and especially vulnerable, food is hamburger or ground meat in general, whether it's ground beef, turkey, chicken, or other meat. Since ground meat receives more handling or processing than many other meat products, it is exposed to many more common food poisoners, and for this reason it is never recommended to eat it raw or rare. For complete safety, make sure your burger is brown, or at least brownish pink, in the center before serving it, or if you're at a restaurant, before eating it.

For meatloaf, be sure to use a probe thermometer to be sure it cooks all the way through to 170°F, especially if the meatloaf contains pork.

Commercially processed meats, such as hot dogs, bacon, lunch meats, sausage and so on, are processed, and contain preservatives, to pretty much eliminate the possibility of food poisoning microorganism survival, and will last longer than many other meat products. These products can still spoil, though, so pay attention to storage time limits.

Hot dogs and lunch meats will keep in the original vacuum-sealed package for 2 weeks. Once opened, though, you should re-wrap it well, and plan to use the rest in 3-5 days. For best flavor use hot dogs no later than one week after the "sell by" date. Also, watch out for liquid which can form around the hot dogs. If it appears cloudy, it can be a sign of spoilage bacteria and the hot dogs should be thrown out.

Eggs and egg-containing foods, as you should already know, need special care. Always observe hot and cold temperature rules for storage of eggs and egg-rich foods.

For best quality, use whole eggs within the week of purchase, and leftover yolks and whites within 2-4 days. The outside limit for keeping whole eggs in the refrigerator is about 5 weeks, after which they begin to lose quality.

As I have already described, the marinating of meat or poultry products requires special care. You should already know that you need to wash any dishes or utensils used in marinating raw meat or poultry with hot soapy water before using it again. So, what else is there to know about marinating foods safely?

There are many different kinds of marinades out there, but basically a marinade consists of an acidic liquid (wine, lemon juice, or vinegar), spices and oil. Since a marinade consists of an acid and marinating can take several hours, you need to use a tray, or bowl, which won't be affected by acid. Glass, plastic or similar material is recommended. Metal pans or bowls, such as copper, brass, galvanized, or gray enamelware should be avoided, as there is the possibility of the acid in the marinade, or for that matter any acidic food, reacting with the metal forming a possibly poisonous mixture. Look at the label of ingredients of the food or additive to be sure it does not contain an acidic substance, such as lemon juice, vinegar, acetic acid or wine before using a metal pan.

Marinating should always be done in the refrigerator. The acid in the marinade may just be enough to slow bacterial growth without completely stopping it. Also, the marinade may not affect or reach through the entire meat product.

As I mentioned earlier, mayonnaise and salad dressings also contain acid, as well as salt, which help to slow, or retard, bacterial growth on foods. In addition, commercially produced mayonnaise (as well as other products) is made with liquid pasteurized eggs. Even though mayonnaise by itself is considered safe, the food mixed with mayonnaise or salad dressing should still be judged on its own, as if it had not been mixed with mayonnaise. Mayonnaise may increase a food's resistance to bacterial growth only slightly, and may not reach the entire dish, so temperature rules and the 2 hour time limit should still apply, for complete safety.

FOOD POISONING HAZARDS

CANNED FOODS

There are two main questions regarding canned foods at home: Where should they be stored? And for how long?

The best place to store canned foods is a cool, clean, dark place where the temperature is maintained at all times below 85°F. Many canned foods tell you right on the label - which should always be read - to store the unopened can at room temperature (around 70°F) and to promptly refrigerate unused portion in a separate container.

How long you can store canned foods depends mainly on the acid level in the food. Low acid canned foods, such as canned meat and poultry stews, vegetable soups (except tomato), spaghetti (noodle and pasta) products, potatoes, corn, carrots, spinach, beans, beets, peas, and pumpkin can be stored for 2-5 years, if the temperature remains consistent and the container is not dented, cracked or damaged in some other way. High acid canned foods, such as juices - tomato, orange, lemon, lime and grapefruit; tomatoes, grapefruit, pineapple, apples and apple products, mixed fruit, peaches, pears, plums, all berries, pickles, sauerkraut, and foods treated with vinegar-based sauces or dressings, like German potato salad and sauerbraten can be stored in the cabinet for 12-18 months. Many cans may be stamped with a "use by" date on the top or bottom.

You should not store high acid foods for too long because of the possibility of the acid in the food reacting with the metal container, producing a poisonous substance. Of course, metal food containers contain a protective coating to prevent this from occurring. Over longer periods of time, though, the protective coating can be worn away, allowing the metal to become exposed to the acid.

If you maintain a large supply of canned goods for long periods of time, it is a good idea to mark them with the date of purchase and to rotate the older ones to the front and the newer ones to the back. This will give you a better idea of how long canned foods sit in your cabinets before being used, so you won't store them past the recommended time limit.

Even though the USDA recommends 2-5 years and 12-18 months, others have recommended that, for the overall safest, highest possible quality (good color, flavor, appearance) you should completely rotate or use up and replace your entire stock of canned foods, both high and low acid foods, every 6 months. This time limit should also include most paper- and plastic-wrapped dry foods as well.

SPECIAL PRECAUTIONS FOR HOME CANNED FOODS

Since botulism food poisoning is much more common in home canned foods, you should boil all home canned foods before serving. Bring the food to a rapid boil which will bring out the bad odors which some botulinum bacteria produce. If the food smells all right, lower the heat and continue boiling the food, covered, for 10 minutes for high-acid foods, and 20 minutes for low-acid foods. This long boiling will destroy any *botulinum* toxin. Complete the long boiling period before tasting for quality or adding seasoning. If the spoiled odor appears or the food is foaming, or looks odd, throw it out without tasting it.

Chapter 5

Reporting Food Poisonings and Violations

Hopefully, after reading the book you now know what to look for and what to do to avoid food-borne illness. You should be able to greatly reduce your chances of getting food poisoning. There is, though, still a possibility, though remote, that you and your family could get food poisoning, despite your best efforts. What should you do if this happens?

STEP I: ACCURATE DIAGNOSIS

First, you should try to confirm that your illness is a possible food poisoning, not just the flu or some similar illness. Remember that the flu is customarily respiratory (like a cold with aches). If diarrhea is your most severe symptom then chances are your illness is caused by something you ate. The two most common food poisoning bacteria, *salmonella* and *staphylococcus aureas*, both have diarrhea and vomiting as their main symptoms. You should be able to tell the difference between the symptoms of food poisoning and the flu by the speed with which the symptoms develop. Flu symptoms usually develop slowly, over a day or two, while the symptoms of food poisoning develop relatively rapidly, within a matter of hours.

Staphylococcus aureas produces a toxin which causes the illness, and will most likely cause more immediate violent spasms throughout the digestive tract and vomiting or vomiting and diarrhea at the same time. This usually occurs 2 to 6 hours, and occasionally 30 minutes to 12 hours, after eating the suspect food.

Salmonella symptoms include headache, rumbling in the bowels, diarrhea and sometimes fever and vomiting, occurring between 6 to 72 hours, usually 12 to 36 hours, after ingesting the bacteria. See the chart in the appendix for other common food poisoning microorganisms and their characteristic symptoms.

Another clue to whether you have experienced a food poisoning is if you were not the only one to become ill. Although this does not happen every time, in many cases more than one person will have become sick from eating the same food and may experience the same or similar symptoms at the same time. Someone may or may not become ill from eating the same thing you did, but if they did and their symptoms are similar, then there is a much greater possibility that you were both food poisoned.

STEP II: EFFECTIVE TREATMENT

The next thing to do, once you've concluded that you probably have a food-borne illness, is to treat your symptoms. If you're only mildly ill, then treat your symptoms much like the flu. Take in much more clear liquids than normal, including water, tea, apple juice, bouillon, or ginger ale to replace lost fluids and you should probably also consult your doctor.

If the symptoms are severe, or if the victim is quite young, elderly or already has a chronic illness, you should definitely have the victim seek medical attention right away. Remember that these groups of people are more likely to have more severe reactions (including death) than others do to food-borne illness.

If you consumed a toxic chemical substance or a foreign object, such as an insect or other bug, or a different type of organism, such as a fungus, mold, yeast or virus, your symptoms could range from vomiting and diarrhea, to a possible allergic reaction, to blood in the stool, or even hepatitis symptoms and more. All of these are very serious and you should see your doctor right away.

STEP III: REPORTING THE INCIDENT

The final thing you want to think about now is reporting the possible food poisoning to your local health department. There are basically three situations in which you should notify your health department when you believe you may have been food poisoned:

1) You ate the suspect food at a large gathering, such as an occasional event;
2) The food is from a restaurant, deli, street vendor catering truck, or other commercial or institutional kitchen; or

3) The suspect food is a commercial product which may have already caused illness or is changed or contaminated in some way which you believe could cause illness.

FOOD POISONING HAZARDS

Try to have the following information ready before you phone in a complaint regarding food poisoning:

1. Your name, address and day time phone number.

2. A brief explanation of the problem: Where did you eat the suspect food? How many other people ate it? Was it a private or public gathering? When (approximate time and date) did this occur?

3. If you ate the food at a restaurant, what is the name and address, and date you ate there?

4. Be ready to give symptoms and the amount of time, in hours, between eating the suspected food and previous meals and the time you first started feeling the symptoms.

5. Try to give a listing of your previous few meals in addition to telling them what food you believe made you ill. It's possible that you could be blaming your illness on the wrong meal.

6. If you've been to a doctor or hospital, they may ask for the doctor's name and phone number who treated you. The doctor's office or hospital may also report your illness to the health department. Check with them if they have already done so.

7. If the suspect food is a commercial product, have the container in hand so you can refer to it while you're on the phone.

8. Try to remember when and where you bought the product. The name and location of the store will help.

9. By law, the container itself must have the manufacturer's name and address, so look for it somewhere on the label.

10. On meat and poultry products, look at the USDA inspection

stamp for the official plant or establishment number. On red meats, you may see something like "Est 38", and on poultry products "P-42". The number identifies the processing plant where the product was made. This information can be very important in tracing a problem to its roots.

OTHER STEPS TO TAKE

It is also a good idea to seal the product in a plastic bag marked "Danger", especially in the case of a possible botulism contamination. To avoid leakage, sit it on a paper plate and refrigerate it on a high shelf, out of reach of children. A health official may want to examine it later.

For reporting any violations you observed at a restaurant, catering truck, street vendor, market or other commercial food facility, be ready with the name, address and date you observed the violation and give a brief explanation of what you observed. Also, be ready to give your name, address and phone number, which will remain confidential, so that the health inspector can contact you after an inspection has been made, in order to let you know what was observed and what kind of action was taken.

WHERE TO FIND HELP

If you have any questions regarding any food products safety or proper handling or anything in general regarding food sanitation and safety, don't be afraid to look up and call your local health department. They are usually listed in the local government pages at the front of your phone book. Or call the USDA's Meat and Poultry Hot Line at 1 (800) 535-4555, or write to: The Meat and Poultry Hot Line, USDA-FSIS, Rm.

FOOD POISONING HAZARDS

1165-S, Washington, DC 20250. If any of these sources can't answer your question they should refer you to someone who can. Also, there are numerous articles and books in your library which cover food-borne illness, food technology, sanitation and more.

Afterword

I hope this book has served its purpose, to inform you of the hazards that are present without scaring you to the point that you will never be able to enjoy another meal. The information I have shared with you can be very useful in improving your chances of staying healthy and increasing your confidence that where and what you choose to eat are safe and healthy choices for yourself and those you love.

I hope you will feel free to write to me at M & C Publishing, 8121 Manchester Blvd., #594A, Los Angeles, CA 90293 with any comments, criticisms or corrections you may have, as well as any experiences you may have had that would add to what I have outlined in this book. I would be happy to hear from you and share whatever information that might advance the cause of public health.

If you would like to purchase more copies of this book, please use the order form provided at the back of the book.

Appendix A

Index of Useful Terms

A

B

C

H

hair	12, 32
ham	93
hamburger	103-104
handwashing	32, 42, 43, 88
hats	12
health departments	45
health of food handlers	14
health permits	48
heating lamps	40
hepatitis	28

- See also Chart,
Appendix C

home canned foods	107

hot dog carts
(See street vendors)

hot water	44

I

ice cream trucks
(See street vendors)

insects	14, 16-18, 36

(See also vermin)

J

jewelry	13

K

kitchen
- restaurant	11-19
- home	87-107

L

labels	62

licenses (See health permits)
lunch meats	101

M

makeup	13
marinating	104-105
mayonnaise	105
meat	27-30

meat and seafood markets
65-72

mice (See rodents, vermin)
milk	37-38
mold	100-102

money and food
handling 12-13

O

occasional events	73

Appendix B

Solutions to Pictorial Puzzles

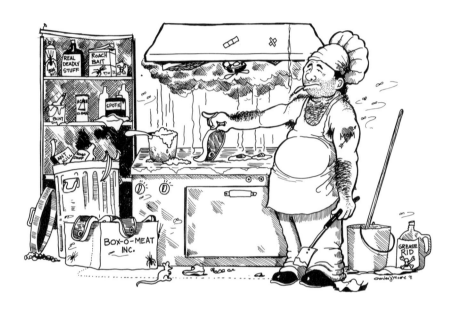

1. The ventilation system or hood should be in good working order and be sufficiently strong enough to remove gases, odors, steam, grease, smoke, etc.

2. Handling food with your hands, with or without gloves, especially meats or other potentially hazardous foods during the cooking process is not a good practice. Hands are a source of both direct contamination and cross contamination if not washed thoroughly and frequently

3. Smoking or other tobacco use can not be allowed during food preparation or utensil washing. nor in food, utensil or equipment storage areas.

4. Flies, 5. Cockroaches, and 6. Mice are all vermin, as are any other insects and are a definite potential hazard to your health.

7. Grease or other food particles accumulated on the stove or other equipment can attract and maintain vermin and microorganisms.

8. Food and food containers should not be stored directly on the floor. The floor can be a source of contamination, especially if a sewage backup occurs.

9. Watch out for food, especially hazardous foods, that are stored at room temperature.

10. Chemicals and other hazardous substances must be stored in separate areas, away from food preparation and storage areas and away from utensil washing and storage areas.

11. Trash containers in a kitchen should have a plastic trash bag liner and not be overflowing. Also, the container must be easy to clean, made of either metal or durable plastic, and leakproof.

12. Trash, food wastes or water should not be accumulated on the floor. During busy times of the day a restaurant may accumulate trash or other wastes on the floor, but it is usually easy to tell the difference between not cleaning the floor during the day and neglecting to do so for a few days in a row.

13. Mops and other cleaning equipment and chemicals must be stored in a separate area or room away from food preparation and storage areas or utensil storage and washing areas.

14. A cook or food handler must wear adequate and clean, preferably white outer garments and/or apron. Body hair and sweat must be blocked from contaminating food or food contact surfaces.

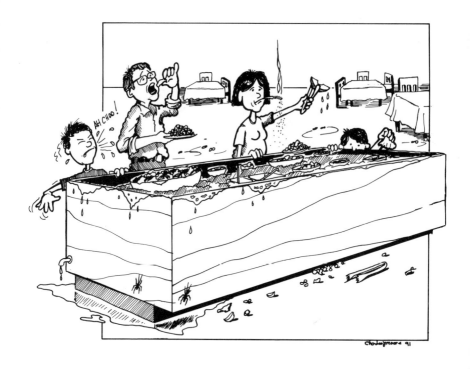

1. The floor area must be kept clean to prevent vermin and microorganism growth.

2. Utensils that have fallen onto the floor must be taken away to be washed and sanitized. Also, each food displayed for self-service should be provided with a utensil with a handle.

3. Water leaking onto the floor from a salad bar or buffet can also attract and maintain vermin and microorganisms.

4. The lack of sneeze guards or other types of protective covering over the exposed foods allows people to contaminate the food by 5. sneezing or 6. smoking.

125

7. When adults or children eat or grab food with their hands at a salad bar or buffet they may ne contaminating food for the rest of us. Although this is sometimes difficult for the management or employees to control, there should be one or more employees overseeing the salad bar and immediately reminding customers to discontinue or avoid any actions that are a potential hazard to others.

8. Flies
9. Cockroaches   Vermin - Need I say more?

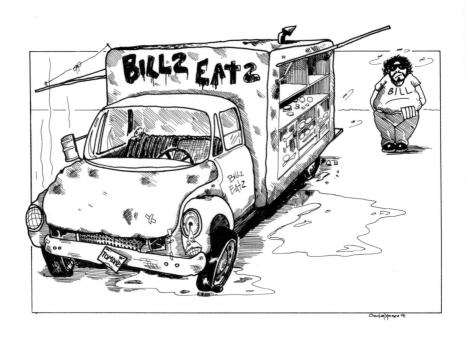

1. The truck itself should be kept in good structural condition.

2. A trash container should be provided for customers to use, to keep trash off the ground.

3. The truck should not be leaking water or purposely draining waste water onto the ground.

4. The business name, address and phone number must be easily readable and posted on both sides of the truck.

5. Flies should not be found near a catering truck.

6. A public health permit with identifying information and an expiration date must be posted in a conspicuous place.

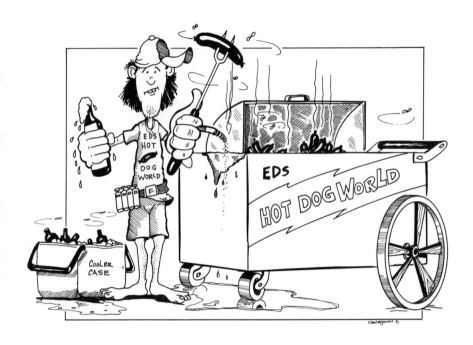

1. Employee smoking is just as hazardous outdoors as it is inside a kitchen.

2. Employees must wear a hair restraint that is adequate for securing or confining all of their hair.

3. Flies must be kept away from any food cart.

4. Water leaking from cart, though it may not directly affect the food, can attract vermin, birds or other animals.

5. No food or beverages can be stored in, displayed or served from any place, such as this cooler case, other than the cart or vehicle itself.

6. An easily readable address and phone number must be posted on at least one side of the cart.

7. The food compartment must be sufficiently large enough to permit food assembly and service operations and must be provided with a tightly fitted closure which is kept closed to protect the interior from dust, debris and vermin.

8. A public health permit must be posted in a conspicuous place and must have such information as the business name, owner and operator's name, some type of vehicle identification number and an expiration date. The lack of this permit, which is different from a business license, could very well indicate that this cart or vehicle has never been inspected and therefore never been approved to operate.

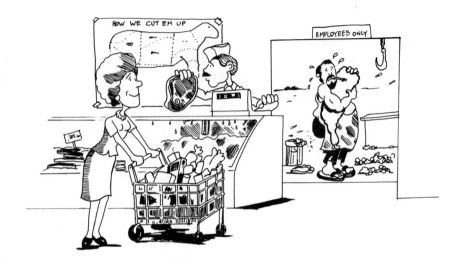

1. The display refrigerator should not be dripping condensation or other waste water onto the food directly below. Condensate water can be potentially hazardous.

2. Employees serving or selling unpackaged meat or other foods to customers must use tongs or other implements rather than their hands.

3. Hair restraints or nets must be worn by all employees.

4. Employee smoking is always a hazard.

5. Employees must wear adequate and clean outer garments or aprons.

6. The floor area must be kept exceptionally clean. Meat scraps should be cleaned up immediately after processing.

7. Flies are always a potential hazard to your health.

8. The trash can, just as in any restaurant, should be easily cleaned, with a plastic bag liner and must not be overflowing.

9. Food handlers should be wearing adequately protective shoes for their own safety as well as for the customers' health.

ORDER FORM

Please send me ____ copies of FIGHTING BACK at $15.95 per book plus sales tax and shipping to:

Your Name or Company Name _____

Address _____

City _____ State _____ ZIP _____

Sales Tax: Please add 7.25% ($1.16 per book) for books shipped to a California address.

Shipping: Please add $2.00 for the first book and $.75 for each additional book. For UPS Second Day delivery, add $5.00 per book.

_____ Books (at $15.95 each) $ _____

Shipping $ _____

Sales Tax (California deliveries only)   + $ _____

Total amount enclosed $ _____

Payment: Check or money order, made out to:
          "M & C Publishing"

Mail this form to: M & C Publishing
                           8121 Manchester Blvd., #594A
                           Los Angeles, CA 90293